W9-BYR-748

Byrne's NEW Standard Book of POOL and BILLIARDS

Also by Robert Byrne

Byrne's Treasury of Trick Shots in Pool and Billiards

Byrne's Advanced Technique in Pool and Billiards

Byrne's Book of Great Pool Stories

Byrne's Wonderful World of Pool and Billiards

Byrne's NEW Standard Book of POOL and BILLIARDS

ROBERT BYRNE

794.73
By
c.1

A Harvest Original
Harcourt Brace & Company
San Diego New York London

Author's note: Because the games of pool and billiards deserve a textbook that is not only comprehensive but completely accurate, I invite corrections, suggestions, and comments from readers for use with credit in future editions. Write to me in care of the publisher: Harcourt Brace & Company, Trade Publishers, 525 B Street, San Diego, CA 92101.

Copyright © 1998, 1987, 1978 by Robert Byrne

All rights reserved. No part of this publication may be reproduced or transmitted in any form or by any means, electronic or mechanical, including photocopy, recording, or any information storage and retrieval system, without permission in writing from the publisher.

Requests for permission to make copies of any part of the work should be mailed to: Permissions Department, Harcourt Brace & Company, 6277 Sea Harbor Drive, Orlando, Florida 32887-6777.

Library of Congress Cataloging-in-Publication Data
Byrne, Robert, 1930–
    Byrne's new standard book of pool and billiards/Robert Byrne.—1st ed.
      p.   cm.
    Rev. ed. of: Byrne's standard book of pool and billiards. © 1987.
    Includes bibliographical references and indexes.
    ISBN 0-15-100325-4 (hardcover).—ISBN 0-15-600554-9 (pbk.)
    1. Pool (Game) 2. Billiards. I. Byrne, Robert, 1930– Byrne's standard book of pool and billiards. II. Title.
    GV891.B96 1998
    794.7′3—dc21   98-14656

Text set in Garamond 3
Designed by Susan Shankin

Printed in the United States of America
First edition
E D C B A

Dedicated with thanks to

Bob Jewett

for twenty-five years

of good advice

contents

7. Practice methods 103

8. Miscellaneous inside stuff 115

2. Twenty ball-first patterns   251

3. Seventeen rail-first patterns   263

4. Diamond systems   273

5. Extensions, variations, extremes, and guidelines   301

6. Fifteen draw, spin, time, and kiss-back shots   321

7. Playing safe, ducking kisses, and getting position   333

8. Fifty selected shots from master play   359

preface

Welcome to the twentieth-anniversary edition! Book One—Pool is almost a third larger than before, with hundreds of revisions and additions. Four chapters are new—those on eight-ball strategy, nine-ball strategy, trick shots, and collecting. Scattered through the text are references to videotapes and other books. The appendixes, Where to Go for More Information, were completely rewritten and updated. The aim was to create the most comprehensive and easy-to-use guide to the cue games ever published.

A lot has happened in the world of cue games since the first edition appeared in 1978. Once dominant games like straight pool and three-cushion billiards have lost ground to eight-ball, the game of choice for millions of tavern league players, and nine-ball, the preeminent tournament game.

Despite the inability of male professional players to unite in a single association, the number of major tournaments and prize funds has grown tremendously. In 1978, even in 1988, pro tournaments were fairly scarce; now the magazines need columns to list them. For the first time in memory, the top fifteen or twenty players are making a good living as full-time professionals. In 1996, for example, a dozen players each made more than $50,000 in tournament winnings, to which must be added earnings from commercial endorsements, exhibitions, and lessons. Six made more than $100,000 in prize money alone.

The Women's Professional Billiard Association has been stunningly successful in recent years and has shown how organization and consistency pay off in attracting sponsors and tournament hosts. The players dress well, look good, and stage very attractive events. It is no longer surprising to find as many women as men on annual lists of leading money winners. Vivian Villarreal won $120,000 in 1996, and Allison Fisher topped $75,000 in 1997, not counting endorsement money. In one memorable day in January of 1998, Fisher, in matches covered live on ESPN, won $65,000. Leader in the endorsement sweepstakes is probably Jeanette "The Black Widow" Lee, who knows how to market herself and makes in the neighborhood of $100,000 a year representing such firms as Imperial International (billiard supplies) and McDermott Cue Mfg. Co. Rewards like these, while far smaller than those enjoyed by golf and tennis pros, were only dreamed of in the pool world ten or twenty years ago.

Even the so-called amateurs are doing better than ever. There are several associations and tavern leagues that hold mammoth annual tournaments featuring hundreds of tables, thousands of players, and hundreds of thousands of dollars in prizes.

New rooms continue to open around the country, though not at the rate seen in the early 1990s. The game is more popular on television than ever before, with ESPN, ESPN2, and SportsChannel devoting serious time to pool competitions. In 1996, Steve Mizerak launched a senior tour that has proven to be popular with the fans. Pool has made great inroads in Europe and Asia, and one day soon there may be an international tournament tour.

The annual industry trade show put on by the Billiard Congress of America, usually in Las Vegas in July, requires almost two hundred thousand square feet of floor space to accommodate three hundred vendors and two or three thousand dealers and buyers. Because the BCA show is not open to the public, pro players Allen and Dawn Hopkins started the annual spring Super Billiard Expo in 1992. Held in Valley Forge, Pennsylvania, and open to the public, the show has grown each year and now attracts about a hundred vendors and six or seven thousand visitors.

Forty-five million Americans pick up a cue at least once a year, double the number in 1978, and pool continues to lead golf and tennis as a participant competitive sport. Bowling is still number one, but the gap is narrowing. If the numbers keep mounting, newspapers will eventually have to admit that pool exists and give it some coverage. Mounting numbers, that's what led to the writing of *Byrne's Standard Book of Pool and Billiards* in the first place.

In early 1977, Tom Stewart, then a senior editor at Harcourt Brace Jovanovich, read a report in the *New York Times* about the huge numbers of pool buffs. He had edited a novel of mine, knew I was interested in the game, and wrote to ask if I could come up with a book on how to play. I replied modestly that I was so perfect for the job it made my flesh crawl, for I had been studying the technique, players, history, and lore of the game for twenty years with an intensity that often confounded and dismayed my loved ones. A contract was soon signed, and I threw myself happily into a writing project I thought would take no more than six months. I say "happily" because an obsession I always regarded as a kind of secret vice had suddenly turned into a business proposition.

A year later, in the spring of 1978, I turned in the manuscript and artwork. When I am asked now how long it took to do the book, I say it took a year to write and twenty years to research. My goal from the beginning was to give the game the manual it deserves, at once comprehensive, accurate, and handsome. HBJ came through with a generous format, good paper and binding, and an attractive cover.

The rest is history, as everything is eventually. *Byrne's Standard Book of Pool and Billiards* was embraced by players and continues to enjoy remarkable acceptance. Twenty years after publication it is still selling around a thousand copies a month and has now sold around 250,000 copies.

I've written twenty-one books—six on the game—but none has brought me more satisfaction than this one. The mail alone makes it worthwhile. One reader, faked out by my omniscient tone, wrote to ask if I could recommend a good teacher in southeast Missouri. Another, apparently suffering from writer's block, asked what English he should use on various shots he tried to describe in a series of long-distance telephone calls.

Special thanks to the hundreds of players who have taken the trouble to write and tell me that my work has helped them improve and enjoy the game more.

Believe me, the pleasure has been all mine.

Robert Byrne
April 1998
Dubuque, Iowa

acknowledgments

My thanks to Lee Simon, proprietor of Buffalo Billiards in Cotati, California, and the earlier Novato Billiards in Novato, California. Without the education I received in those institutions over the past twenty years, writing this revised, expanded edition would have been a nearly impossible task. Also essential were the hundreds of comrades, competitors, and correspondents in the pool and billiard worlds who challenged my theories, deepened my understanding of the game's many layers, and, on occasion, proved their points by beating my brains out on the green cloth.

For permission to reproduce the covers of *Billard, mit dem offiziellen Teil des Billardsportverbandes Österreich,* thanks to Heinrich Weingartner of Vienna, the "Mr. Billiards" of Austria.

For permission to reproduce the Julia Roberts cover of *International Billard* (which is sensational in color), thanks to Bertrand Le Port, directeur de la redaction, Tamaris Presse, Nogent sur Marne, France.

Thanks to Elaine Duillo for permission to reproduce the illustration she did for *The Wedding Gamble,* by Cait Logan, published in 1996 by Dell.

Thanks to Tim Bieber of Mr. Big Productions, Chicago, for permission to reproduce the photograph *What's the Best Shot?*

Thanks to St. Martin's Press for permission to reproduce the cover of *The Howard Hughes Affair* by Stuart Kaminsky (illustration by Joel Iskowitz, 1979).

Finally, thanks to my editor at Harcourt Brace, Christa Malone, for her diligence and good humor.

introduction

This book is devoted to two great games, pool, which is growing in popularity all over the world, and three-cushion billiards, the secrets of which were not revealed until this book appeared in 1978. Very few games are "great." A game is great, in my view, only if it can be played happily by a sane person of at least average intelligence for several hours a day for fifty years. Both pool and billiards qualify.

By the word *pool* I mean what the industry, in its attempt to sanitize its history, persists in calling "pocket billiards." I have never heard a pool player call the game anything but pool. No player ever says to another, "Would you care to play a game of fourteen point one continuous pocket billiards?" He says, "Let's play straight pool." By *billiards* I mean that family of carom games played on tables without pockets, which are more common than pool tables in most non-English-speaking countries. Billiards is also taken to mean all forms of cue games, as in "the billiard industry."

Snooker, a game played on a six-by-twelve-foot table with narrow pockets and small balls, is not discussed directly. Much of what is said about the technique of playing pool applies equally well to snooker.

Byrne's New Standard Book of Pool and Billiards focuses mainly on teaching the reader how to play, how to play better, and how to play still better. (I ask the indulgence of women and left-handers for assuming that the reader is a right-handed man. The goal is to simplify the text, not shut out and ignore more than half the world's population.) Little space is devoted to the history of the game, as long and colorful as it is; to the champions and hustlers, as amusing and appalling as some of them are; or to stories of my own exploits as a player, most of which are false. Here we will stick to technique, tactics, and strategy. The book is a course of instruction that will take you from kindergarten to graduate school. At the end you'll have an understanding of physics and English not taught at conventional institutions of higher learning.

Don't quit your day job, however, unless you are phenomenally gifted. Play the game for fun, as a hobby, not for a living and not for your health. While tournament play is exciting and sometimes returns your entry fee, it's no substitute for a job that permits you to call in sick and still get paid. Pool hustling as a career choice is even worse because it's dangerous. All that secondhand smoke and high-fat finger food! If you know a good player who is tempted by pool hustling, introduce him at once to a career guidance counselor, a psychotherapist, or a surgeon who does lobotomies. Petty thievery is a more profitable job than pool hustling, which it resembles, requires far less talent and training, and is equally devoid of promise.

That playing pool and billiards is somehow good for your health is a tack long taken by manufacturers and industry flacks. I don't think the game is *harmful* to health; it is on recreational rather than medical grounds that I recommend it. There surely were more invigorating physical things to do even in 1881, when *Modern Billiards* first appeared. That great book, a gold mine for historians, especially in its expanded later editions, quoted a Dr. Marcy, "the well-known American physician," as follows:

> One of the pleasantest and easiest means of regaining and retaining health is to introduce into private houses a billiard table, and to present it to the entire family as a means of daily exercise. . . . The most indolent and stupid will, by practice, soon acquire a fondness for the game; and the improvement in the sanitary condition of those who habitually indulge in it will commend it in the strongest manner to the heads of families. We also advocate the game of billiards in families from a *moral* as well as a *sanitary* point of view. Young America is naturally "frisky" . . . and fond of excitement and fun. . . . Give them a billiard table so that body and mind can be amused and invigorated, and the attractions and pleasures of home will be superior to those beyond its boundaries.

As Ned Polsky pointed out in his fascinating book on the sociology of the poolhall subculture, *Hustlers, Beats, and Others* (Aldine, Chicago, 1967; Carroll & Graf, New York, 1998), the billiard world has always been divided into two main streams, the public room on the one hand and private clubs and home on the other, with little leakage between them. Tournament promoters not so long ago made players dress in tuxedos to blur the distinction, but without ever really fooling anybody. While my own career has been conducted almost entirely in public facilities—Walt and Hank's in Boulder, Colorado, when I was pursuing an engineering degree, Palace Billiards in San Francisco when I was editing a trade journal, and Harry's in Novato, California, until it closed in 1986—I think I would be better suited temperamentally to the quieter confines of a paneled clubroom or a stately mansion, where liveried retainers would fetch my tea. My feelings, in fact, for the game and for the book you are now reading are precisely those expressed by H. W. Collender in *Modern Billiards* more than a hundred years ago:

> The game of billiards has reached such a high degree of popularity that the billiard table has become a requisite in every well-furnished modern household, and to play a fine game is regarded as one of the accomplishments of every well-educated gentleman. To reach the proficiency of the great experts is not, of course, easily attainable, but to become a good amateur player is not an extravagant ambition. It is within the province of everyone gifted with ordinary natural abilities and aided by a good textbook, which will guide him step by step to master the strokes usually presenting themselves in a game, to reach a degree of skill which will entitle him to rank as an accomplished player. The present treatise, besides answering such a purpose, will be found to be the most perfect ever offered to the public.

While I welcome constructive criticism for possible incorporation in future editions, please send complaints and whining to the Dead Letter Office, United States Postal Service, Washington, DC.

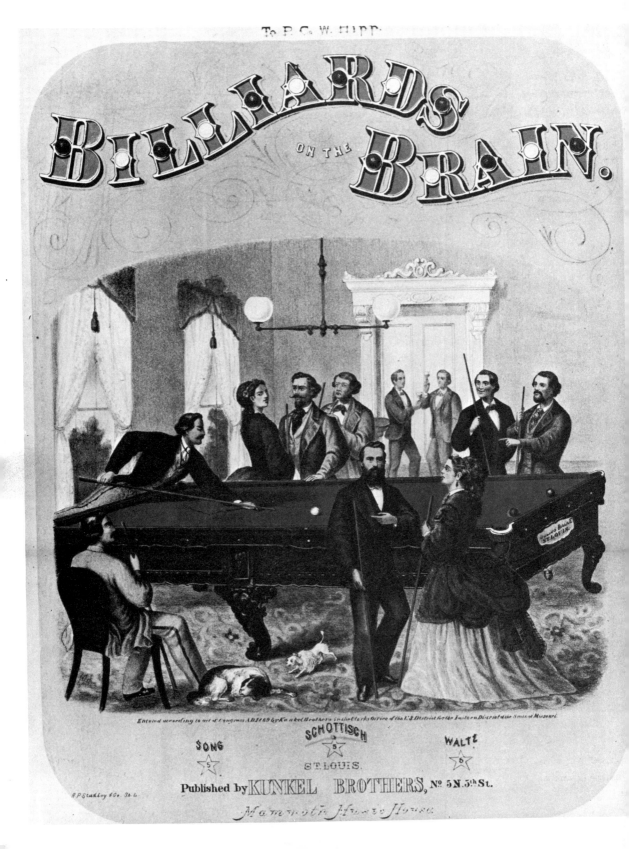

book **1**

POOL

Sheet music published in 1869.
(Byrne Collection)

fundamentals 1

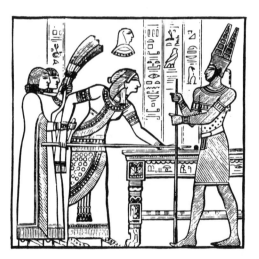

Shakespeare said Cleopatra played;
he was wrong.
(*Modern Billiards,* 1881)

The table

A family can have a lot of fun on a department store pool table costing only a few hundred dollars. The fake wood composition bed, unpredictable cushions, and generally flimsy construction permit luck to overwhelm skill. Shoot hard and the balls might land on the floor; shoot softly and they'll roll like eggs. A cheap table will frustrate even the best player's intentions, and there is always the amusing possibility that it will collapse completely.

Such a game can be fun as long as the equipment holds up, especially for kids, but it isn't pool. Pool, properly so called, requires a table costing considerably more than a few hundred dollars, unless you get lucky on the secondhand market. The table has to be at least seven feet long (pros insist on nine); otherwise the game becomes trivial, like marbles. It has to be solid enough so that if somebody bumps it, the balls won't rearrange themselves. It has to have a slate bed because slate doesn't warp, lasts forever, and is rigid enough to resist acting as a trampoline. Slate can take the punishment that children and drunks dish out.

Slate, unfortunately, is heavy, which means that furniture designed to hold it must be heavy, too, and well made. You can't buy a piece of heavy, well-made furniture for less than, say, $1,200, not if it is supposed to be a pool table of decent size and quality. For something good, think $2,500. Top-of-the-line models boasting superior craftsmanship, materials, and styling run between $3,000 and $7,000, depending on the maker. If you have exquisite taste and plenty of money, ask your local billiard supply dealer to show you an antique or a replica of an antique—they cost from $10,000 to $50,000, but they look terrific in a game room.

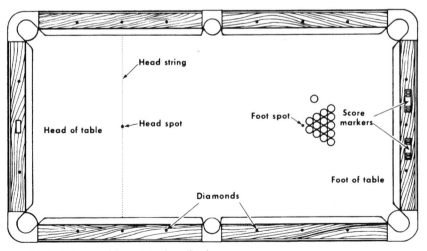

The field of play and how it is described

Three thousand dollars isn't out of line when you consider that, after purchase, a fine pool table costs almost nothing to use and will last forever. Aside from cloth and cushions, there is nothing to wear out. Furthermore, a good table retains a substantial resale value, while a table that was junk to begin with is destined only for the dump, and soon.

The cue

It is a pleasure to report that as the twentieth century ends and the twenty-first begins, you can still buy a decent one-piece pool cue for less than thirty dollars. It will last a certain number of years without warping or splitting. It won't have inlays of exotic woods and mother-of-pearl, but if pointed in the right direction and thrust suddenly forward, it will knock balls into pockets with soul-satisfying regularity, beyond which not a great deal should be asked of a cue.

If you want to carry a cue from place to place without accidentally prodding people, you'll need one that comes apart in the middle, which adds about fifty dollars to the price. If you also want well-seasoned wood, superior workmanship, and a leather, twine, or linen grip, prepare to pay at least two or three hundred dollars. Add 50 percent for a cue custom built to your specifications. Beyond, say, five hundred dollars, you are buying inlay work and ornamentation, which can easily add a thousand dollars to the price. Some of the high-end cues are extraordinarily beautiful and can give you tremendous pride of ownership, if not a better pool game. Quality of play is probably more affected by the tip than the cue. Give a pro player a broomstick with a good tip on it and he'll not only make some remarkable shots, he'll sweep the joint out afterward.

A cue should be between fifty-seven and fifty-eight inches long, provided you have a normal wingspan and are between sixty-six and seventy-six inches long yourself. Leaving aside the special needs of tiny people as well as normal-sized people trying to cope with miniature home tables, it can be said that a pool cue should weigh between sixteen and twenty-one ounces. The diameter of the tip should be between eleven and thirteen millimeters. The "right" size and weight are whatever feel best in your hands.

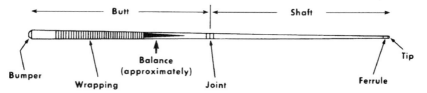

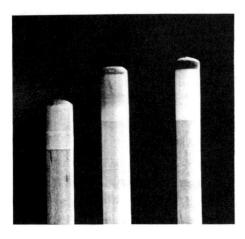

Tips on cues—The tip at the far left is bad because it is too thin and lacks resilience at the edges. It should be replaced. The tip in the center is too flat but can be rounded off with sandpaper. At the right is a properly groomed tip with a curvature approximating that of a nickel. Keep overhangs sanded off.

If you are shopping for a cue, talk to a dealer that specializes in billiard supplies or the proprietor of a billiard room that has cues for sale. Some sporting goods stores and department stores sell cues, but on such premises it is hard to find clerks who are sensitive to the nuances of weight, size, balance, taper, flexibility, and craftsmanship. Usually all they will know about a cue is how to record its sale. Shun a cue that breaks down into more than two parts, has a tip that screws on, is painted in festive colors, or is made in Taiwan. Made in Japan is OK; the Adam line, made there, is one of the best.

Satisfaction is almost guaranteed if you go to a cuemaker and have him custom build one matched to your arms, fingers, and intentions. The cost, about $300 to $500, will not be much more than top-of-the-line models available off the shelf, and you'll have a fine piece of personal woodwork that will last a lifetime.

It's easy to make a cue last a lifetime. Don't boil it or freeze it in the trunk of a car. Don't lean it against a wall for years. If you lose a game to a complete idiot, hit the edge of the table in anger with something other than your cue. Don't swordfight with it, even in jest. Never poke anything with it other than cueballs. Don't store it near kindling. Withhold it from relatives, neighbors, pets, and offspring.

A dirty cue and a sweaty hand tend not to slide smoothly over one another. If you turn to talcum powder for relief, apply it sparingly to the crotch of the thumb. Wipe the excess off your palms before touching the cloth of the table or you'll mess it up, much to the irritation of people like myself. Next time your cue feels sticky, clean the shaft with a damp cloth and dry it thoroughly, then do the same to your hands, adding soap to taste. If your hands sweat a lot, keep a dry cloth within reach. If the shaft still sticks to your skin, clean it with one of the many creams and solutions designed for the purpose. Sandpaper coarser than

Don't use scouring pads to combat stickiness—they're too rough. Better are the new abrasive papers that are finer than the finest sandpaper. See your billiard dealer.

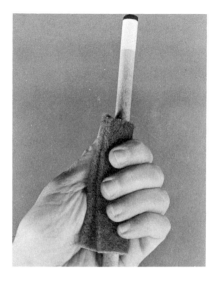

#2000 and kitchen scouring pads like Scotch Brite, unless they are used with an extremely soft touch, take off so much wood that your cue will, over time, be turned into a long toothpick. Better for removing films of grease and grit are the very fine abrasive papers available at billiard stores.

The tip

Most top players like a medium-hard-to-hard tip rather than a soft one, even though it has to be roughened once in a while to make sure it will hold chalk. The shape or contour of the tip is very important. There is no excuse for tolerating a misshapen tip, as it takes only a minute to make it right. The tip will last longer and will work best if it is exactly the same diameter as the end of the cue. There shouldn't be the slightest evidence of overhang at any point—if there is, stand the cue with the tip down on a flat surface, press down, and trim off the excess with a sharp knife. Smooth off the knife marks with fine sandpaper. Harden and burnish the edges of the tip by first moistening them, then wrapping the end of the cue inside a matchbook cover or piece of leather and rubbing rapidly up and down. An optional cosmetic finale is to paint the sides of the tip with a black felt pen.

Don't try to play with a tip that is flat or nearly flat. Take a piece of medium sandpaper, fold it over enough times to provide a stiff backing, and round the tip off to the approximate curvature of a nickel.

Putting a new tip on a cue takes some time and fussing but isn't difficult. Start with the best tips you can get, as the cost is negligible compared to other

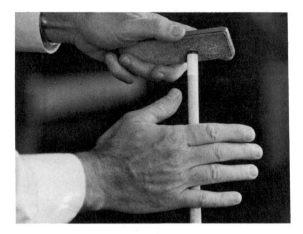

A hard tip is better than a soft one, but it may need to be roughened once in a while so it will hold chalk. I roll the cue on a small block of wood with two grades of sandpaper glued to it.

ways you waste money. With a knife and sandpaper, remove the dried glue and what's left of the old tip from the end of the cue. The flat surface of the ferrule must remain flat, so be careful not to round off the edges. Select a tip that is slightly larger than the ferrule or precisely the same size and roughen the bottom of it with sandpaper. Apply a thin coating of glue to the ferrule and the tip. Elmer's white glue is fine, but don't use epoxy or any of the superglues because they are too hard to scrape off next time around. Center the tip on the ferrule and press down on it with your thumb until it will stay in place by itself. Carefully stand the cue in a corner, as vertically as possible, with the tip down. In the morning, trim off any overhang and shape the top of the tip. If you have more cues to fix than corners, buy a tipping kit from a billiard supply dealer or farm the job out to the guy who does it for the local poolhall.

A new tip may flatten slightly during the course of play and may have to be retrimmed and reshaped. It may also become so hard and shiny that it won't hold chalk, in which case it must be roughened lightly with sandpaper, a file, or any one of a number of gadgets called scuffers designed for the purpose. Some tips are so hard they need scuffing several times during a game.

Miscues are usually caused by a loose bridge or a crooked stroke, but scowling at the tip to divert suspicion from yourself is de rigueur.

The chalk

A thin coating of chalk increases the friction between the tip and the cueball. You can't apply spin to the cueball with any assurance unless the tip is chalked. Chalking up after every shot is not overdoing it.

Brush chalk across the tip frequently with light side-to-side strokes. Don't roll the cue into the chalk as if trying to bore a hole. Chalking up after every shot is cheap insurance against miscues.

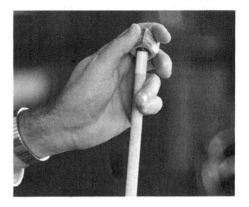

When applying chalk, don't spin the cue into it with the flat of your hand. Hold the cue still and use a rocking motion of the cube. Look at the tip to make sure it is coated completely; if not, touch it up with light brush strokes.

If you want to be regarded as thoughtless or if you are deliberately trying to irk your opponent, leave the chalk on the rail so that he has to walk all the way around the table to get it. If there is only one piece, put it absentmindedly in your pocket. I advise against secretly spitting in it in the hope of causing your opponent to miscue because that ploy has been known to lead to compound fractures of the thumbs.

A habit deplored by refined pool players everywhere is putting the chalk on the rail upside down. The resulting smudges get on the cloth and on everybody's hands and clothes. Always lay the chalk down *exposed side up.* If you don't, onlookers may conclude that you tend toward the slovenly in other areas of life as well.

A point of etiquette: Don't pick up the chalk when you miss because that is when your opponent is reaching for it.

Not all chalk is good chalk. Good chalk is hard and fine-grained. Good chalk costs more than coarse, soft chalk, but only a little.

Cloth, cushions, and balls

Billiard cloth can be fast or slow; cushions and balls can be dead or lively. Because there aren't many varieties to choose from and because styling isn't a factor, the shopper has to remember only one simple rule: You get what you pay for.

Balls once were made of ivory; then a shortage of elephants drove the price too high. Today's cast phenolic resin balls are superior to ivory because they are cheaper, truer, and longer lasting.

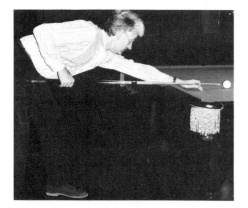

My stance is more erect than most, typical of players who play a lot of three-cushion billiards. Most top pool pros have a lower aiming crouch than shown in the photo and a longer bridge. For the classic pendulum style, only the fore-arm moves during warm-up strokes while the elbow remains fixed in space directly above the cue. For maximum force, move the right hand back six inches from your normal shooting position.

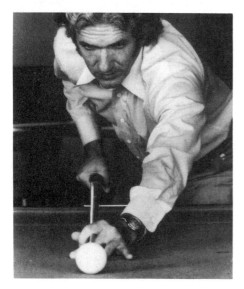

Like the great majority of players, I stand with my dominant eye directly over the cue so that I can aim it like a rifle. A few center their chins over the cue. The photo was taken in 1977, before I dyed my hair gray.

The first nonivory balls were invented in 1868 and were made of celluloid. Their tendency to spark and even explode on impact lent a festive atmosphere to the game.

The stance

There is no one correct stance. When you are bent over the table aiming a shot, part of your weight will be on your left foot, part on your right foot, and a little on your left hand. The proportions vary from one player to the next, as does the placement and attitude of the legs, arms, and head. Some expert players keep both knees straight and spread their legs widely; others keep their feet fairly close to-gether and flex both knees. You might feel comfortable with only your left knee

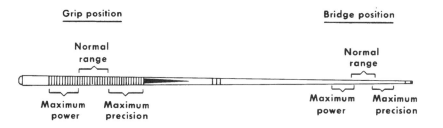

bent and most of your weight forward. Some players stand rather erect; others crouch so low their chins graze the cue. They are always comfortably and solidly balanced, though, and most (not quite all) have one eye directly over the cue so they can aim it like a rifle or an arrow. If your stance conforms to these guidelines, you can ignore those who would have you arrange yourself differently.

You should adopt the same stance for every shot that provides easy access to the cueball. To that end I recommend keeping the left arm perfectly straight, thus eliminating one variable.

The grip

Don't clench the cue like a baseball bat with the thumb and all the fingers tightly encircling it, and don't hold it delicately at the fingertips like a fop with a tea-spoon. Most players enclose it lightly but firmly with the thumb and forefinger. Another finger or two can lightly rest on the underside. At the limit of the back-swing, just the thumb and forefinger touch the cue; at the end of the follow-through, all of the fingers grip it. Don't lay the thumb along the top of the cue because that blocks proper wrist action. Don't lock the wrist.

The position of the right hand can vary somewhat from shot to shot. For a soft shot requiring maximum precision in speed and English, one for which the right "touch" or "feel" is critical, move the right hand forward to the front of the wrapping, a few inches behind the balance. For shots requiring maximum force, position the hand at the rear of the wrapping. On most shots the right hand should be six inches or so behind the balance. When you are ready to hit the cueball, move the cue tip to a point halfway from the cueball to your bridge hand. Is your forearm now pointing straight down? It should be, or close to it.

Please do not write to me in care of the publisher to point out that two of the greatest players of all time, Willie Hoppe and Ralph Greenleaf, violated these and other precepts. There are professionals in every sport with peculiar styles. Talent, years of heavy practice, and a fanatic will to win can compensate for any number of flaws in technique. Those of us who have better things to do than play pool all the time had best stick to orthodox methods.

The bridge

Simply laying the cue across the left hand in the groove formed by the thumb and forefinger provides an unobstructed view of the shaft and is OK for shots that can be stroked softly, that require no English or a long reach. Beginners who use such a bridge—as the left-hand support for the cue is called—on every shot shouldn't be ridiculed too much for it. The open or V-bridge is serviceable, and beginners have enough to worry about without forcing them into uncomfortable and distracting hand positions. Later, though, they'll have to find a satisfactory closed bridge with the forefinger encircling the shaft—it's the best insurance against miscues and the only way to apply spin with security.

Holding the cue properly is one of dozens of critical factors involved in learning to play pool and billiards acceptably. Without a good bridge you can hardly expect to advance beyond the klutz class. Study the photographs and note that

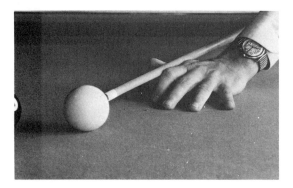

The open or V-bridge is OK for shots requiring no English, little force, or a long reach, and for games with small balls, like snooker. The groove between the thumb and forefinger must be narrow enough to keep the cue from wobbling. Keep the heel of the hand on the cloth.

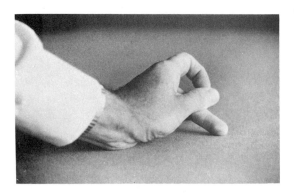

The closed bridge should be learned early on. Lay the hand flat on the table with the fingers spread. Slide the tip of the middle finger across the cloth to the right under the forefinger and form an X with the middle of the thumb. Curl the forefinger until the tip touches the thumb, as in the photograph. If necessary to achieve perfect snugness, push the tip of the forefinger between the thumb and middle finger. Keep the heel of the hand down and the middle, ring, and little fingers spread.

Follow bridge—To hit the cueball above center, form a higher bridge without raising the heel of the hand off the table.

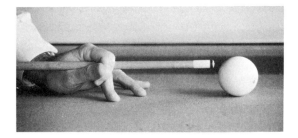

Draw bridge—To hit the cueball below center, lower the thumb and forefinger; *don't raise the butt of the cue.* Keep the cue level unless you want the cueball to jump or curve.

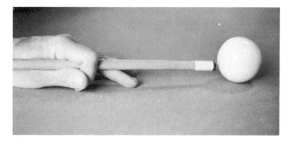

The follow-through should be at least as long as the backswing, preferably longer, provided there are no obstacles. Think of hitting *through* the cueball. The cue should continue in a perfectly straight line until it slows down and stops naturally at the end of the stroke. Don't stop the cue short, even on draw shots.

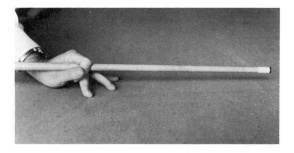

Don't do this! A terrible habit that must be broken at once is letting go of the cue before completing the follow-through. The previous photograph—*that's* how it should look. Hang on and stay down. Don't raise the cue, move the hand, jerk the head, or straighten the body.

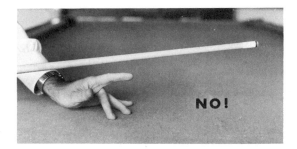

NO!

there is a satisfactory hand position for even the most difficult situations. Strive for snugness without impeding the back and forth motion of the cue.

It's an advantage to be able to shoot left-handed in positions that would otherwise require the use of the mechanical bridge—also called the rake and the crutch. Using the rake requires a right-arm position that restricts warm-up stroking and makes it harder to closely control speed and English. If you *must* use the rake, hold the butt of it on the table with the left hand to make sure the bridge end doesn't move, align the cue so that the rear of it points at your chin, hold your right forearm roughly parallel to the bed of the table, and use short warm-up strokes with a little extra wrist action. Be prepared to snatch the rake off the table upon hitting the cueball to avoid a foul.

Stroke

Before bending over, decide on what shot to shoot, where the object ball must be struck, and what speed and English are needed to make the cueball do what you want it to. Don't be vague. Make specific decisions—otherwise the outcome of the shot will teach you nothing. If you change your mind in any significant way after crouching, straighten up and start over.

Once you feel you know the line of aim, assume a stance that is comfortable, form a firm bridge, and plant your left hand on the table. Make sure your head is directly over the cue and the cue is free to move smoothly back and forth.

Position the cue tip close to the cueball—less than half an inch—so that when you finally "pull the trigger" you won't have to lunge. Adjust your stance, grip, and bridge if necessary to get on the line of aim. (I assume here and throughout the book that you want to play as well as your natural ability permits you to instead of simply to pass the time.)

Watch top players and you'll see that they don't all use the same stroke. There are several acceptable styles; you'll have to find the one that suits you best. I'll

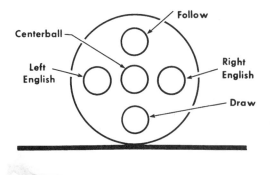

In this book "English" means sidespin and sidespin only. Hitting the cueball below center is called "draw" and not "low English." Hitting it above center is called "follow" and not "high English." Combinations are called high left, low right, and so forth.

Rail bridge used by almost every top player allows the cue to stay as low and level as possible. The cue is pinched between the forefinger and middle finger with extra guidance provided by the left thumb, which is alongside the cue rather than under it. The right way to form most bridges involving a rail is to lay the cue down first, then form the hand around it.

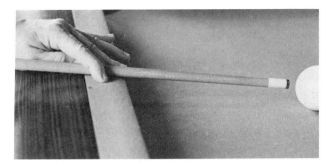

Rail bridge at an angle differs from standard rail bridge only in that the forefinger curls inward slightly to keep the cue pressed against the side of the thumb.

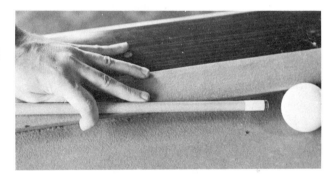

Rail bridge parallel to the cushion—now the forefinger is looped around the cue and the thumb has room to extend under it. The tips of the thumb and middle finger are on the bed cloth.

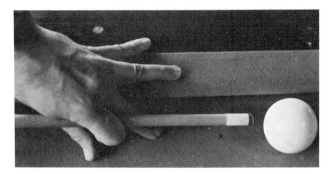

Don't do this, please! Don't form a standard bridge on the rail in this position because it forces you to shoot down on the cueball. Keep the cue level unless you are intending to make the cueball jump or curve.

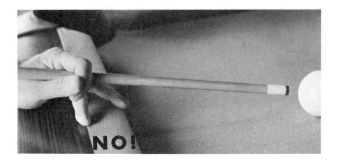

describe in detail a way of stroking that works well with newcomers and also with good players trying to escape from a slump.

After you are in the aiming crouch, move the cue back and forth a few times to get the feel of how fast it will have to be brought forward to give the cueball the proper speed. Stop the tip at the cueball and make sure the cue is on the correct line of aim. Stroke once or twice more to see if the cue stays on line and make whatever fine adjustments are necessary. Once you are satisfied that the cueball will hit the object ball neither too thick nor too thin, take two more rhythmic strokes and pull the trigger, following through evenly. At the end of the follow-through, the tip should be close to or on the cloth; never allow the cue to swerve or rise. Leave your hand on the table for a second or two.

Some players don't stop the cue to aim; they do it during the warm-up strokes. Others use a slow, controlled final backswing. Others pause for one beat before pulling the trigger when the tip is at the hand. A few bring the tip back only halfway to the hand on the final backswing. I call these four strokes the classic, the drawstring, the hesitation, and the poke. Try them all.

A good stroke is hard to teach because it is partly instinctive and only partly learned. If you feel yours leaves something to be desired, study an expert and try to imitate the way he handles the cue when addressing the cueball; better yet, ask him to give you a lesson. In the meantime, review the following checklist, an amalgam of my own convictions larded with the tested wisdom of yesteryear:

1. Decide on what to do before bending over.
2. Plant your left hand closer to the cueball for soft shots than for hard ones.
3. Grip the butt of the cue farther forward for soft shots than for hard ones.
4. "Place the cuetip nearly against the cueball and exactly at the point you intend to strike it." (J. F. B. McCleery, *The McCleery Method of Billiard Playing, Containing One Hundred Elegant Engravings,* Payot, Upham & Co., San Francisco, 1889)
5. Make sure your bridge is snug.
6. Keep the cue as level as possible at all times, even on draw shots, unless you want to make the cueball curve or jump.
7. Take a few warm-up strokes to get the feel of the force required and to refine the aim.
8. Strive for warm-up strokes that are smooth, easy, silky, straight, graceful, flowing, measured, authoritative, and solid, not hurried, crooked, "pokey and inelegant." (Arthur Peall, *All About Billiards,* Ward, Lock & Co., London, 1925)

Draw shot off the rail—To hit the cueball below center from this position, you must raise the butt of the cue. Slip the thumb under if there is enough room. To avoid unintentional massé (curve) action, be careful not to hit the cueball right or left of center.

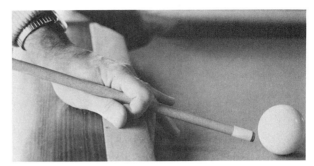

Frozen ball rail bridge is difficult because there is no place to plant the heel of the hand and still provide room for warm-up strokes. One method is to brace the hand as firmly as possible against the edge of the table with the fingertips. Elevate the cue slightly to guard against miscuing over the top of the ball. Make sure to hit the cueball without sidespin.

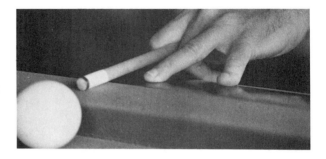

Shooting over a ball is a terrible problem for most beginners. The trick is to use an open bridge, place the hand close to the obstructing ball, elevate the cue just enough for clearance, and hit the cueball without a trace of English.

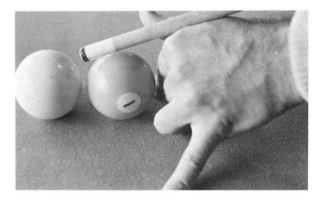

Shooting over a ball—another view. Note how middle fingers are folded out of the way but still provide some support. Most of the weight is supported by the extended little finger and forefinger.

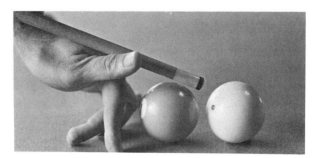

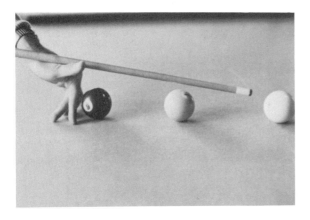

Shooting over two balls is not so tough once you get the hang of the high bridge. Restrict the length of your warm-up strokes in over-the-ball shots to an inch or two. The critical factor is the avoidance of English.

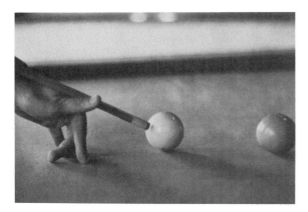

The massé or jump shot—A good angle for those massé or jump shots that are practical under game conditions is about half of 45 degrees. Hit with English, the cueball will curve around the edge of an interfering ball; hit in the center and with some force, the cueball will jump over the edge of the interfering ball. The most common mistake made with both types of shot is shooting too hard.

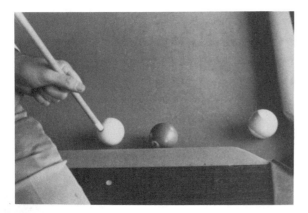

The freehand massé, in which the bridge hand is removed from the table and braced against the body, involves a downward stroke from a steep angle. Astonishing curves are possible, but the shot is so unreliable it is almost never seen in tournament play. (Banking for the object ball or playing safe are saner strategies.) Massé shots are fun to fool around with, though, on somebody else's equipment.

9. Don't worry about your right wrist. Some players use a lot of wrist action, some don't.

10. Take at least three warm-up strokes, but not more than six or eight, except on unusually delicate or difficult shots. "Avoid excessive preliminary fiddling." (Maurice Daly, *Daly's Billiard Book,* A. C. McClurg & Co., Chicago, 1913)

11. Look at the object ball last, not the cueball. In fact, closing your eyes shouldn't affect accuracy very much once you've found the line of aim and grooved your stroke.

12. Hit through the cueball without any feeling of checking your stroke, *even on draw shots.* "Let the ball have that last finishing caress." (Willie Hoppe, *Thirty Years of Billiards,* G. P. Putnam's Sons, New York, 1925)

13. Follow through at least as far as you draw back.

14. Don't try to steer the cueball during the follow-through by swerving the cue tip to one side or the other; try to develop a straight delivery that doesn't veer off toward the side of the English.

15. Hold your body still! Freeze the head and shoulders! The elbow should be motionless during the stroking motions, dropping only at the end of a long follow-through. "Persons who throw their bodies forward after the cue would do well to renounce the game, for that quality totally unfits them for the delicacy of touch and firmness of body, eye, and purpose which are the grand essentials of success." (H. W. Collender, *Modern Billiards,* Trow's Printing and Bookbinding Co., New York, 1881)

16. Keep your bridge hand on the table until the stroke is complete.

17. Don't "baby" the ball. "A good stroke must be made crescendo, that is, increasing in speed until contact. Timidity will cause you to spare the shot, with a resultant foozle." (*Daly's Billiard Book*)

18. Because God hasn't given us the gift of seeing ourselves as others see us, as the Scottish bard Burns discovered well over two hundred years ago ("giftie gie us" is how he put it, if memory serves), entrust this book to a friend while you are practicing and have him criticize your stance, bridge, grip, stroke, and follow-through.

19. When you miss a shot during a game, step away from the table with good grace; redouble your resolve and await your next opportunity without morbid brooding about the shot you missed. "Nobody likes a smart-ass" (Solzhenitsyn), and nobody likes a complainer, either.

20. If you lose, so what? It's only a game, a game as thrilling as skydiving but cheaper and not so hard on the joints. Don't explain to the winner how lousy

you played; congratulate him instead on a fine performance—after all, he beat a terrific player.

21. Because a poor loser is such an ugly spectacle, pursue excellence rather than victory at all costs.

22. Ignore the words of Will Johnston of Peacock Gap, California: "Show me a man who doesn't cheat and I'll show you a man that I can beat."

23. When confronted by a hysterical and possibly homicidal loser, remind him of what the English physician Sir Astley Cooper said: "We should all sleep more soundly if we made it a rule to play billiards an hour or two each evening." (*Modern Billiards*)

Attitude

A surprisingly large part of pool skill is a matter of attitude and concentration. When the pressure is on, the player with the best control of his nerves and emotions has a big advantage.

Try to play with confidence, even if you have little reason for having any. The sooner you act like a good player, the sooner you'll become one. I don't mean you should swagger, pose, brag, and sneer like some of the insufferable clowns you see at tournaments, but I do mean you should cultivate an air of command. When it's your turn to shoot, don't come to the table with your face a mask of fear and indecision; step right up as if everything is under control. Handle the chalk and cue with the illusion of easy familiarity. Survey the mess on the table as if a computer is whirring in your head producing printouts of favorable odds. For your brain *is* like a computer, and if you practice enough, it will begin making decisions for you on an unconscious level about speed, hit, and spin. When that happens, people will begin saying, perhaps even writing, that you have a nice feel for the game.

Acting like a good player even though you are miscast in the role is not so much for the purpose of frightening your opponent as it is for building up a feeling of confidence within yourself. In many areas of life and pool, a confident mental attitude is almost as important for success as luck and cheating. You must be able to make cold-blooded assessments of percentages, but once you decide to try a certain shot it pays to do so with forthrightness and even ebullience. You've got to believe that you can make the shot, that you *will* make it. At the moment of truth there is no room for pessimism. Once you allow yourself to start worrying about how hard the shot is, how poor your chances are of making it, how bad you are going to look if you miss, how embarrassing it will be to lose the game . . .

well, then that exquisite machine you've been fine-tuning is almost sure to belch, backfire, and run off the tracks.

Phrased as an apothegm: Mental control is as important as cueball control.

Reference: Skill at pool depends on solid fundamentals. There is little point in continuing your education until you have a secure grasp of such preliminaries as stance, bridge, grip, and stroke. It's hard to overemphasize their importance, and what I've said here is by no means all that can be said. See the early chapters of *Byrne's Advanced Technique in Pool and Billiards* (Harcourt Brace, 1990) and *Byrne's Wonderful World of Pool and Billiards* (Harcourt Brace, 1996), where a different approach to the subject is taken.

While there is no substitute for the diagrams and depth of detail in books, which can be studied at a pool table or taken to bed, students can speed their progress with the help of videotapes. Dynamic factors like cue speed and stroke rhythm are hard to explain in a book, though easy on a videotape.

Fundamentals are covered in the first section of *Byrne's Standard Video of Pool, Vol. I* (Premiere Home Video, 1987), where, among other things, the classic stroke is examined. In *Rack 'em Up* (Premiere Home Video, 1996) the four general types of stroke are demonstrated in both real time and slow motion.

centerball shots 2

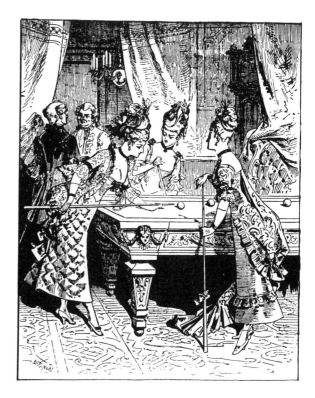

In the court of French king Louis XV.
(*Modern Billiards*, 1881)

Players argue about the percentage, but something in the neighborhood of half the shots in a typical game of pool require no English—that is, the cueball can be hit exactly in the middle. Striking the cueball off-center to make it spin is essential for advanced play, but it increases the chance of miscuing and confronts the shooter with such variables as curve, throw, and squirt, which will be dealt with later.

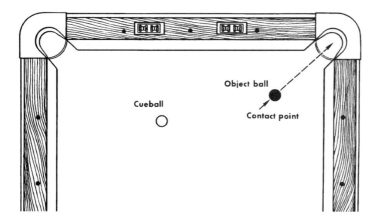

1 Lining up a shot

There are several ways to aim a cut shot. The one that makes the most sense to newcomers and the one described here is called "the ghost-ball method." Start by visualizing where the cueball must contact the object ball to send it into the pocket. With exceptions to be dealt with later, the contact point is directly opposite the pocket. Warning: The contact point is not the point at which you aim the cueball. See Diagram 2.

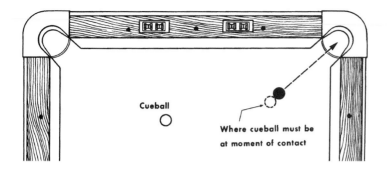

Cueball

Where cueball must be
at moment of contact

2 At the moment of impact

The second step is to imagine the cueball at the moment of impact with the contact point. The imaginary ball is the so-called ghost ball. A line from the pocket passes through the centers of the object ball and the ghost ball.

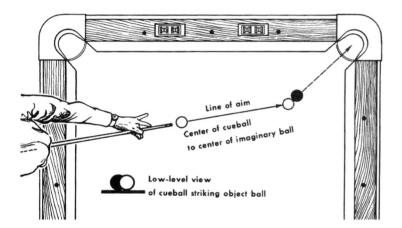

Line of aim

Center of cueball
to center of imaginary ball

Low-level view
of cueball striking object ball

3 Where to aim

Third, shoot the cueball straight at the center of the ghost ball, which sends the object ball into the pocket. It works no matter where the cueball is at the start. If the cueball crosses the center of the ghost ball, the shot must make. The aiming process becomes automatic with practice.

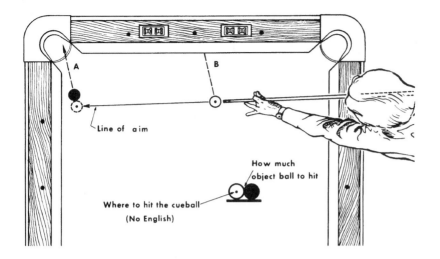

Line of aim

How much
object ball to hit

Where to hit the cueball
(No English)

4 Another aiming aid

The dashed ball represents the cueball at the moment of contact. To make thin cuts like this, the cueball must just barely brush the side of the object ball, as shown in the enlarged inset. Considerable speed must be used because only a small part of the cueball's energy will be transmitted to the object ball. If after diligent practice you still have trouble judging cut shots, try locating the contact point on both the object ball and the cueball. Making the shot is then a matter of driving the two contact points together. In the diagram, line B is parallel to desired object ball path A. Where B intersects the rim of the cueball is the cueball contact point.

● ● ●

While the geometric aiming method described in Diagrams 1–4 is useful at first, you will soon discover that you must hit the object ball slightly thinner than indicated. The reason is that the phenomenon of "throw," discussed in Section 6, affects cut shots as well as combinations. When a cueball hits an object ball on a cut shot, friction between the balls causes the object ball to be thrown slightly off line. Chalk or dirt on the balls makes the effect more pronounced. Throw on cut shots can be eliminated by using "outside" English, which enables the cueball to roll off the object ball like a cogwheel instead of rubbing against it.

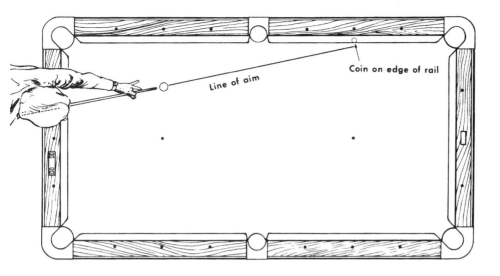

Line of aim

Coin on edge of rail

5 Making a coin jump off the rail

Here's a shot that drives home the idea that the contact point is not the aiming point. Put a coin on the rail so part of it overhangs the nose of the cushion. Challenge a friend to hit the coin with the cueball, starting from the shallow angle of approach in the diagram. The secret is to aim the cueball well past the coin so that the left edge of it hits the coin or the rubber under the coin. A good hit makes the coin jump. Aiming directly at the coin is futile, yet that's what most beginners will do.

Reference: From a different cueball position, it's not difficult to make the coin jump into a glass. For a demonstration, see *Byrne's Standard Video of Trick Shots, Vol. III.*

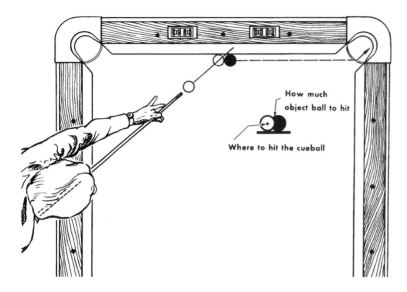

How much
object ball to hit

Where to hit the cueball

6 Running a ball down a rail

If a ball is frozen to a rail and is only a foot or two away from a corner pocket, the shot can be aimed as if the rail didn't exist—aim through the center of the ghost ball as you would on an ordinary cut shot. If the margin of error is small, however, as it is when you must run the ball down a rail past the side pocket, the secret of success is to hit the rail a hair before hitting the ball. The rail-first hit allows the cueball to sink into the rubber before contacting the object ball, resulting in the slightly thinner hit needed on cut shots as explained in Section 6, Throw Shots. I must repeat that the cueball hits the rail just *a hair* before the object ball. The difference between hitting the rail first and hitting the ball and rail simultaneously is so slight it can't be detected with the naked eye when the balls are in motion. When aiming, I suggest lining up for a simultaneous rail-ball contact, then shading the line of aim just slightly away from the object ball.

Reference: You'll find an entire chapter devoted to the subject of running balls down rails in *Byrne's Advanced Technique.*

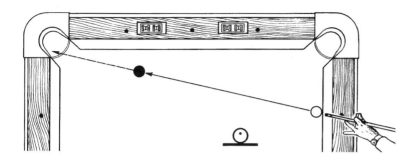

7 Shooting off the rail

Shooting off the rail into a cueball on the cushion isn't easy because there is no way to make a solid bridge and still have room to stroke. Because you must elevate the butt of the cue an inch or two to minimize the risk of miscuing over the top of the cueball, it is vital to hit the cueball on the vertical axis. If the tip contacts the cueball even the slightest bit to one side or the other, it will curve off line (the massé effect) on its way to the object ball. When the shot is straight in as diagrammed, shoot softly enough to keep the cueball from following the object ball into the pocket.

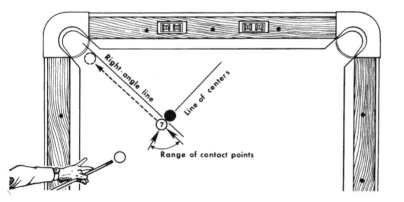

8 The kiss shot

Count your blessings when the balls line up like this. The 7 will go in if it is hit anywhere between the two arrows, a generous margin of error. Without the black ball, the cut would be impossible. Here's how to tell if the shot is "on": Imagine a line through the centers of the two object balls (the line of centers) and a line at right angles to it between them (the right-angle line). The edge of the 7-ball will travel along the right-angle line. The shot is easiest to calculate when the balls are frozen (touching one another).

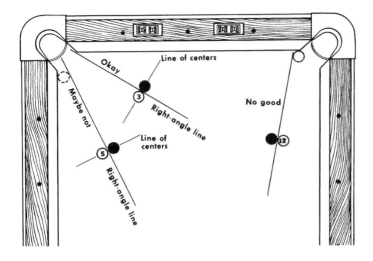

9 Kiss shots—on, off, and maybe

The 3-ball can be made off the black ball because its right edge (looking toward the pocket), traveling along the right-angle line, clears the corner of the rail. The 5-ball shot is unclear because projecting the right edge of the 5-ball along the right-angle line indicates that the left edge of the ball might hit the rail. The 12-ball is a sure miss because the right-angle line falls too far to the left of the pocket.

Ways of forcing an object ball off the right-angle line will be described in Section 6.

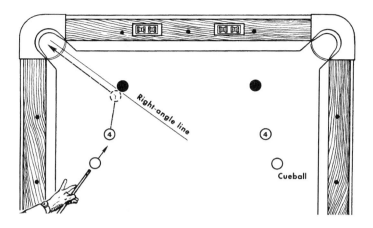

10 Calculating a carom shot

Consider the position on the right side of the diagram, which can arise in infinite variety. Can the 4-ball be made off the black ball? Yes. To find out what must be done, imagine a line from the pocket to the edge of the black ball as shown on the left side of the diagram, where a mirror image of the shot is laid out. That is the right-angle line. The dashed ball is where the 4-ball must be at the moment of impact so that the line of centers between the two balls is perpendicular to the right-angle line. To make the shot, drive the center of the 4-ball toward the center of the imaginary ball.

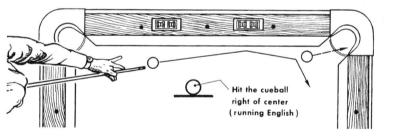

11 Playing off the rail

If the object ball is close to a pocket as well as close to a rail, it is almost as easy to knock it in by playing the cueball off the rail, an approach especially useful for playing position when the shot is straight in. "Running English" (spin that makes the cueball go faster after touching a rail) is not essential but makes the angle easier to estimate.

    NOTE: As in all the diagrams in this book, the line represents the path the center of the cueball takes, which is why it does not touch the rail or the object ball.

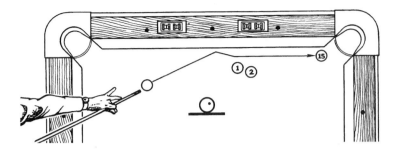

12 A rail-first carom shot

Don't overlook shots of this type, which are often quite easy. The diagram shows an application in a game of rotation. The 15-ball can't be made by driving the 1-ball into it because the 2 is in the way. The cueball can do the job by bouncing off the rail into the 1. Running English isn't essential, but it helps.

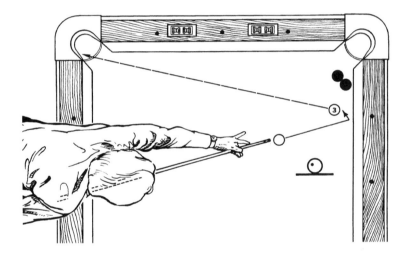

13 A rail-first bank shot

The black balls obstruct the right-hand corner pocket and the 3-ball can't be banked because the cueball would get in the way. A possible solution to the problem is to send the cueball into the rail behind the 3. This is never an easy shot but is sometimes the best chance.

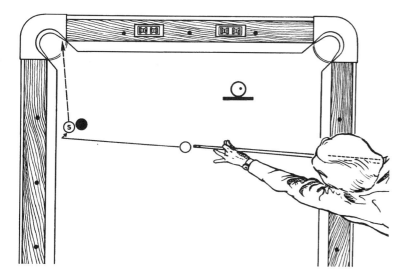

14 A rail-first kiss-off shot

Slicing the 5-ball into the corner pocket is difficult because of the extremely thin hit required. The shot is easy coming from the opposite direction, thanks to the favorable position of the black ball, so play the cueball off the rail. Before shooting, of course, make sure the shot is "on" by the method explained in Diagram 8. English isn't needed, but some is shown for this particular angle to make sure the cueball rebounds into the 5 squarely enough.

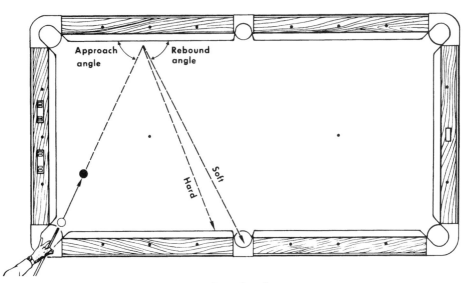

15 At last, the truth about bank shots

It's hard to think of a subject about which the American people have been more con- sistently misinformed than bank shots. Time and time again they have been told to "divide the angle," but what does that mean exactly and how is it done? Inexplica- bly, the greatest player in history has it all wrong in his two otherwise splendid small books on the game (*Willie Mosconi on Pocket Billiards,* Crown Publishers, New York, 1948, and *Winning Pocket Billiards,* Crown, 1965). The balls are usually in a position that makes the use of arithmetic messy. Further, since a pool ball bouncing off a cush- ion is not a light ray bouncing off a mirror, it is only roughly true that the angle of incidence equals the angle of reflection. At shallow angles the rebound angle is less even without running English. Still further, speed and English have almost as much effect on the angle of rebound as does the angle of approach.

Diagrammed is a position of rare purity. Both the cueball and the object ball are on a line running from the corner pocket to the midpoint of the opposite rail. The angle is divided! If the object ball is propelled softly along the dashed line, there is a good chance that it will bank across the table and vanish into the side pocket. However! Hit the ball hard and it will come short, as it would if there were right- hand English on the cueball. And how would you find the correct contact point on the opposite rail if the object ball were a few inches to the left to begin with?

The harsh truth is that professional players use judgment rather than geom- etry on bank shots. Properly blending the angle, the speed, and the English is more a matter of art than science. The only way to get good at bank shots is to shoot them till they come out of your ears.

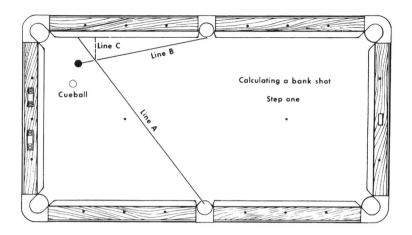

16 Calculating a bank shot—step one

For readers who are more analytical than artistic, here's a way of finding the theoretical contact point on the rail for bank shots. Put the tip of your cue on the rail directly opposite the object ball and lay it on the table on line A, which leads to the target pocket. Imagine line B from the object ball to the other side pocket. From the intersection of A and B drop a perpendicular to the rail, line C. Where C hits the rail is the contact point.

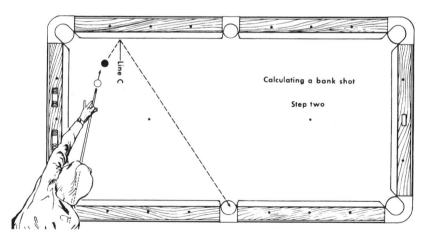

17 Calculating a bank shot—step two

Now comes the hard part—making the object ball hit the calculated point on the rail. Shoot softly. A little left-hand English may help.

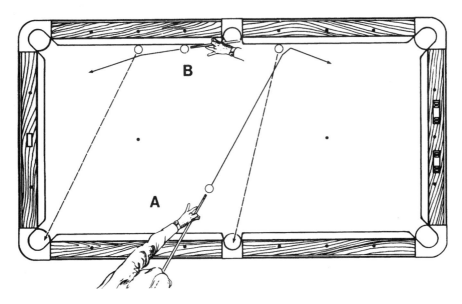

18 Two practice banks to keep you busy

Shot A can be made with the cueball even farther to the left. In shot B the balls are frozen to the rail and one diamond apart—any closer together and the shot becomes nearly impossible.

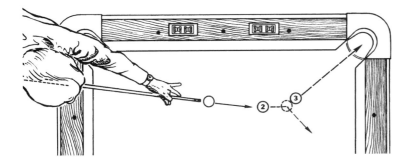

19 A two-ball combination

Combination shots are usually far harder to make than single-ball shots of the same length because the contact point on the second ball presents a smaller target than the pocket. In figuring the diagrammed shot, imagine where the 2-ball must be at the moment of impact, then knock the 2-ball through the center of the imaginary ball.

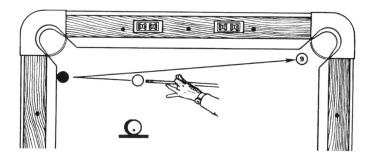

20 The double-kiss or kiss-back shot

A shot like this is called a double-kiss or a kiss-back. By hitting the black ball a hair to the right of center, the cueball will be thrown back in the direction of the 9-ball. Shots of this type are sometimes overlooked even by experienced players unless they also play billiards. The angle is not particularly difficult to judge if the first ball is frozen to the cushion and the cueball is directly opposite it as shown. Hit the cueball low for good action. Subtleties are shown in Diagram 30 at the end of the next section.

Reference: For more on banking, see The Truth about Bank Shots in *Byrne's Advanced Technique.* It is helpful to know that the angle a ball rebounds off a cushion depends partly on whether or not the ball has natural roll (no slippage between the ball and the cloth) or is sliding when it hits the cushion. A surprising and mysterious way to show the difference is diagrammed in Facts about Follow, Skidding, and Banks in *Byrne's Advanced Technique* and is demonstrated on Volume V of my videotape series, *Power Pool Workout.*

Did you know that if a ball is located precisely in the center of the table it is possible to double and triple bank it in the side? The secret is revealed in The Truth about Bank Shots in *Advanced Technique* and demonstrated in the *Power Pool Workout* video.

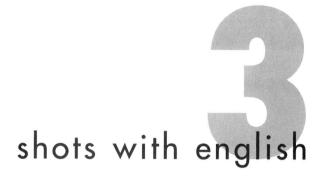

shots with english

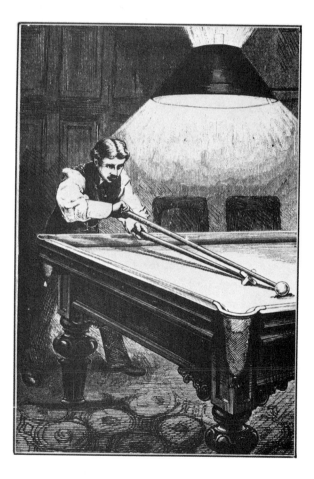

(Byrne Collection)

Mingaud and the discovery of English

The contribution to human happiness made by Captain Mingaud of the French infantry has gone unrecognized. No sidewalk boasts his handprint, nor any Hall of Fame his bust. He sits astride no granite horse in any public park. In or about 1807 in Paris, France, when people there and in England were still pushing billiard balls around with blunt wooden poles as if they were so many shuffleboard pucks, Mingaud unleashed a new invention, the leather cue tip, thereby changing the course of recreational history. For a time he stood alone in all the world in his ability to make a cueball spin. He could make it curve so spookily that suspicions must have been raised about the ownership of his soul. The latter part of his life was devoted to giving exhibitions that dazzled the crude and the effete alike.

Thanks to Captain Mingaud . . . and to others, like Bartley and Carr of Bath, England, who gave us chalk around 1820, John Thurston of London, who introduced slate for table beds a few years later, and the American, Michael Phelan, who redesigned the cushions using vulcanized rubber in 1856 . . . the game was imbued with such a range of subtlety and richness that it metamorphosed from an idle pastime into a thing of beauty and a splendid challenge to human powers of coordination, concentration, and creativity. There's enough to it now to fascinate the finest minds among us. Master the practical applications of a spinning cueball and you'll not only have a trade to fall back on, you'll be an object of wonder to the children of every land.

More on Mingaud and other curious lore about the game's beginnings can be found in *William Hendricks' History of Billiards* (Roxana, Illinois, 1974). A good recap of the game's history is the late Clem Trainer's piece in the fifth and later editions of *The Encyclopedia of Sports* (A. S. Barnes and Co., New York). For historical works with plenty of four-color illustrations, see *Pool,* by Mike Shamos (Mallard Press, New York, 1991), *The Illustrated Encyclopedia of Billiards,* by Mike Shamos (Lyons & Burford, New York, 1993), and the monumental *The Billiard Encyclopedia,* by Victor Stein and Paul Rubino (Blue Book Publications, Minneapolis, Minnesota, 1996). The latter book is reviewed in *Byrne's Wonderful World.*

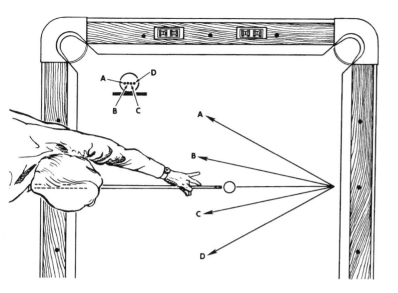

21 English off a rail

If the cue tip contacts the cueball off-center, a sidespin component is added to the normal forward roll. The farther from the vertical axis it's hit, the more it spins. Applications are myriad. Place the cueball as shown and shoot straight into the side rail. Note the change in the rebound angle as you hit the cueball farther and farther from the center. Even a beginner should be able to bank the ball into the corner pocket with a little practice. To get the maximum effect, chalk the tip completely, hit the ball halfway from the center to the edge, and use soft speed.

Reference: Halfway from the center to the edge of the cueball is as far as you can go without miscuing when applying maximum follow, draw, or sidespin. If you have access to a file of *Billiards Digest* magazine, see Dr. George Onoda's article in the August 1991 issue on off-center hits and how to use a striped ball as a cueball to practice them. (The edge of the stripe marks the halfway point.) I discuss Onoda's halfway rule with the aid of close-up photography in the video *Power Pool Workout*.

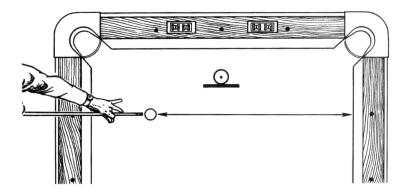

22 How true is your stroke?

It's hard to hit the cueball dead in the middle. To see if you can do it, shoot across the table at right angles. If your stroke and follow-through are straight and if your estimation of a centerball hit is good, the cueball will rebound squarely into the tip of the cue. When you've done it five times in a row, turn 90 degrees and use the full length of the table. Five times in a row the long way requires nearly perfect technique. If you suffer from the common beginner's habit of raising your hand and the cue too soon, practicing this shot will help you break it.

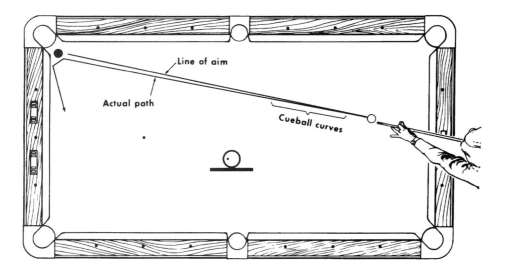

Line of aim

Actual path

Cueball curves

23 Allowing for the curve

Unless your cue is precisely level, sidespin will make the cueball curve. The more sidespin you use, and the more you hit down on the cueball, the more the curve. If you were faced with the diagrammed shot and left English was needed for position on the next shot or to break up a cluster, you would have to aim to hit the object ball full in the face to compensate for the curve. At low speeds, most of the curve takes place in the bracketed area; the harder you shoot the closer to the object ball the bracket moves. On a hard stroke the cueball has no time to curve at all—in fact, it will "squirt" in the opposite direction (see Diagram 108, Curve versus "squirt," at the end of Section 5 in Book Two).

To minimize curve when sidespin must be used, keep the cue as level as possible; one way to do it is to let the butt end graze the rail at the beginning of the warm-up strokes.

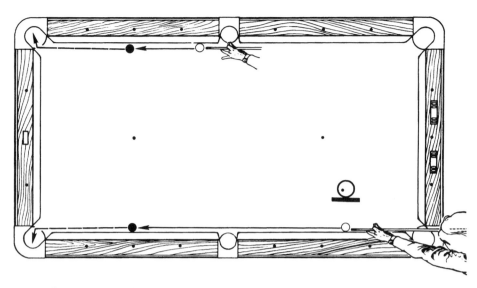

24 Two deceptive shots along the rail

At the bottom of the diagram, both the cueball and the object ball are frozen to the rail with the side pocket between them. The shot can be made with a center-ball hit provided the cueball isn't deflected by the corner of the pocket. To avoid that lamentable possibility, use left English and aim the cueball so that it leaves the rail by the smallest possible fraction of an inch. With a little luck, the English will bring the cueball back to the rail beyond the pocket and hold it there until it hits the object ball. Shoot softly to give the English a chance to work and to avoid following the object ball into the corner.

The shot at the top contains a different pitfall. The black ball is slightly off the rail. Unless the bed cloth is new, a soft hit on the cueball might allow it to become trapped in the groove that is worn along the rail. Shoot hard enough to make sure the cueball travels in a straight line.

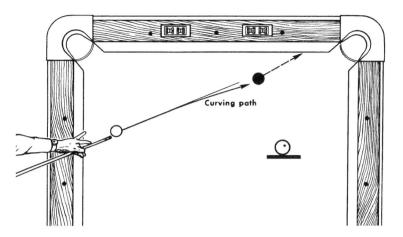

Curving path

25 A frequently missed shot

The shot is not quite straight in. Using high right English and shooting hard for reasons of position make it more difficult than it looks because the cueball will deflect to the left of the line of aim ("squirt") and also curve to the right because of the right spin (assuming you are hitting slightly down on the cueball, which is normal). Avoid sidespin unless you are sure of the shot.

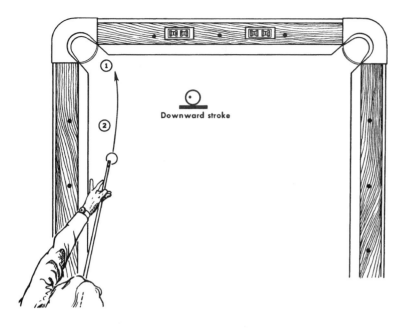

Downward stroke

26 The dreaded massé shot

Sometimes you don't want to minimize the curve by keeping the cue level. Diagrammed is a possible position from a game of rotation, in which the cueball must contact the lowest-numbered ball first. The rest of the balls have been omitted for simplicity. The 1 is hidden behind the 2. In poolroom parlance, the player can't see the 1. Without an easier option, a massé shot can be tried. With the balls placed as shown, it would be necessary to aim downward at an angle of between 30 and 40 degrees with maximum left English. Shoot just hard enough so that the cueball skids past the 2 before breaking to the left. Good luck.

Reference: The massé shot is explained in detail in *Byrne's Advanced Technique* and demonstrated on *Byrne's Standard Video of Pool, Vol. II.*

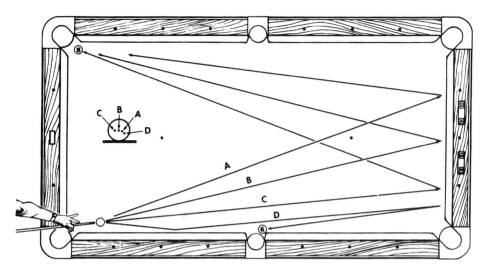

27 More examples of English off a rail

See if you can develop some consistency in banking for the 8-ball along paths A, B, and C. Path A calls for "hold-up" or reverse English (as opposed to running English), so called because cueball speed is reduced, or held up, when it strikes the rail. Another example of hold-up English is illustrated by path D, which intrigues bystanders who have never seen it before. Try it out on your friends and children; it's the kind of shot that might kindle an interest even in the most torpid. Better they be interested in pool than nothing.

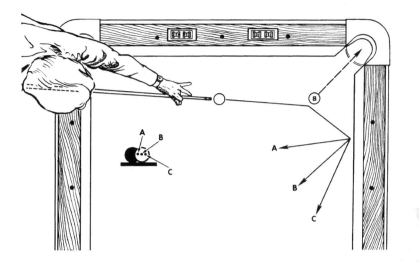

28 English off a ball, then a rail

Hitting the cueball above center (follow) or below center (draw) changes the path the cueball takes after hitting another ball, but sidespin (English) has no appreciable effect. In the cut shot shown, the path from the 8-ball to the rail is the same for left, right, and centerball hits on the cueball. Once the cueball hits the rail, though, provided the speed is the same in each case, the difference is great. When trying to duplicate the diagrammed paths, make sure you don't hit the cueball below center, which will impart draw action and move the contact point on the rail farther to the right.

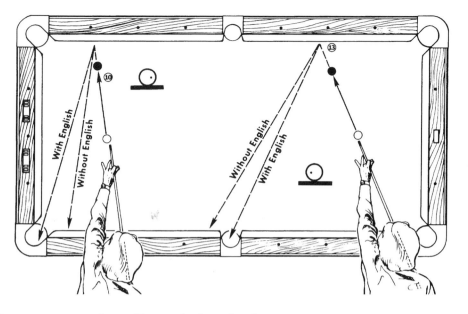

29 How to make off-angle bank shots

A small amount of cueball spin can be transferred to the first object ball. As with meshed cogwheels, the direction the object ball turns is opposite to that of the cueball. Usually, the amount of spin transferred is too trivial to worry about, but on banks it is of crucial importance. Many banks are missed by the unthinking application of English; others can be made that seem impossible.

At the left above, the black ball can't be hit on the right side because of the 10-ball. Hitting the black ball without English will bring it across the table short of the pocket. The shot can be made with right English on the cueball. Shoot softly because high speeds tend to move the rebound angle closer to the perpendicular.

At the right is the opposite problem. The black ball seems destined for a point beyond the side pocket. To make the shot, use left English. The small amount of right English the black picks up will "shorten" the angle. Shooting firmly helps in this case.

Reference: For more on what influences bank shots, check the sources mentioned on page 37.

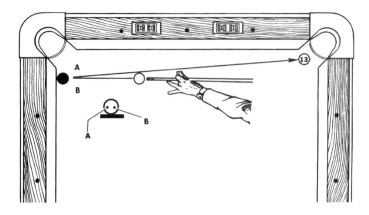

30 A subtlety in the kiss-back shot

Only the best of the best players know that not only can the 13 be pocketed rather easily on a kiss-back shot, but that the final position of the black ball can be influenced as well. Right English sends the black to B; left English sends the black to A. In a game of rotation you might want to leave the black at A so that you can make it easily after the 13. But if the 13 is not so favorably placed, it might be better to leave the black at B to deny your opponent a simple shot if the 13 fails to drop.

Reference: Three of the four three-cushion kiss-back shots diagrammed at the end of Section 6, Book Two, can be applied to pool. Make one in competition and you'll be called a magician.

follow, stop, and deadball shots

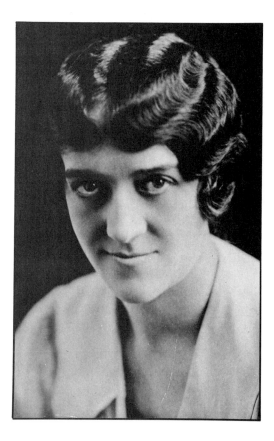

Ruth McGinnis, perhaps the best female
straight pool player in history.
(Byrne Collection)

Hitting the cueball above center on a straight-in shot makes it follow the object ball along the same path, sometimes right into a pocket for a scratch. With experience you can estimate to within a few inches how far the cueball will roll in pursuit of the object ball; the harder you hit it and the higher you hit, the farther it will go. The cueball will follow the object ball for a short distance on soft shots even without above-center cuing. Follow action occurs if the cueball is rolling when it hits the object ball. If it is sliding across the cloth rather than rolling, or if it is turning forward at less than the normal rolling rate, other things occur. We'll discuss follow as well as the other things in this section.

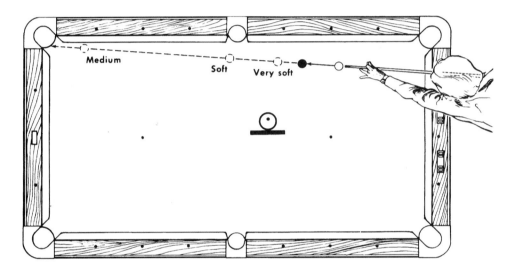

31 Making the cueball follow the object ball

The dashed balls indicate approximately where the cueball will stop when it is struck above center at various speeds. With high follow it would be possible to follow the object ball into the corner without shooting hard.

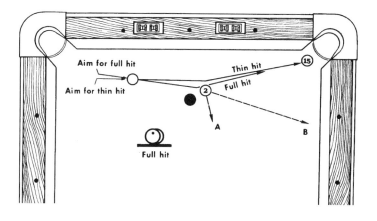

32 The drive versus the cut

Billiard players are routinely faced with the decision of hitting the object ball thick or thin—that is, of driving or cutting the object ball. Pool players, by contrast, often overlook the fact that on many shots they can hit the object ball in two places and still carom the cueball along almost the same path. Diagrammed is a shot from a game of rotation. Most pool players would try to pocket the 15 with a thin carom off the 2, cutting the 2 along path A. (The black ball prevents driving the 2 into the 15.) There might be a positional reason, however, for using follow to "go through" the 2-ball, sending the 2 along path B. Sometimes the thin hit is much the more difficult of the two choices.

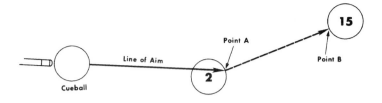

33 How to aim a follow shot

There is an approximate method of finding an aiming point for follow shots like the one in the previous diagram. From point B, where the 15-ball must be struck, imagine a line to the nearest point on the 2-ball, which is point A. To send the cueball through the 2 into the 15, aim at point A with high follow and a soft stroke. The trouble with this system is that it was developed in the last century when there were still plenty of elephants wandering around, which is to say that it works best with ivory balls. Today's phenolic balls require a slightly thicker hit. The system, unfortunately, is usable over a fairly small range of angles and speeds. If you watch for carom shots in games, it's surprising how many you'll find.

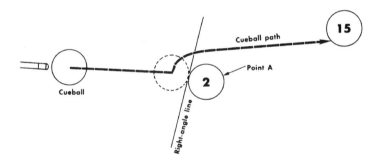

34 What really happens on a follow shot

When the cueball is sent toward point A, it doesn't follow straight through the 2-ball to the 15. What happens is that it first moves along the right angle formed by the 2-ball and the cueball at the moment of impact. The instant the cueball leaves the 2-ball its path is bent forward by the topspin (the curve is a parabola). The harder you hit the cueball—provided you cue it well above center—the wider the curve. See next diagram.

NOTE: Unless interaction among additional balls is involved, as on the break shot, the cueball does not bounce backward before diving forward.

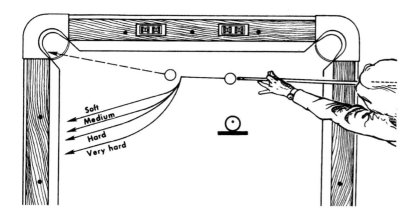

35 How speed affects follow shots

Burn this diagram into your mind. As explained in the last diagram, the harder you hit a follow shot, the flatter the forward curve is. Understanding this action enables the skilled player to make some beautiful shots.

Reference: Because a clear grasp of these curved cueball paths is essential to advanced position play, I urge you to watch *Byrne's Standard Video of Pool, Vol. II,* where they can be seen in both real time and slow motion from an overhead camera.

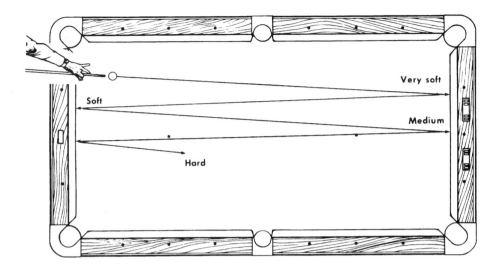

36 Medium speed is three table lengths

On your table the rubber may be dead, the balls dirty and sluggish, and the cloth may have a heavy nap that robs the cueball of its speed. That is your problem. My problem is to give you an idea of what I mean by soft and hard. A soft stroke will carry the cueball the length of the table and back. A hard stroke is good for four table lengths and then some. Except for the break shot in such games as eight-ball, nine-ball, and rotation, it is rarely necessary to hit the cueball hard. Pool properly played requires finesse and foresight rather than power. If you like to slam the balls around without thinking ahead, approaching the game as if it were a kind of demolition derby, we must face the possibility that you and this book are not well suited.

Fast cloth costs more because the nap must be shaved off at the mill, but it is a pleasure to play on. Accuracy and touch replace brute strength. Break the balls on fast cloth and they really spread. Ask your dealer for 860 cloth made by Simonis in Belgium. Stick to coarse, tough cloth if your table might be attacked by roughneck kids.

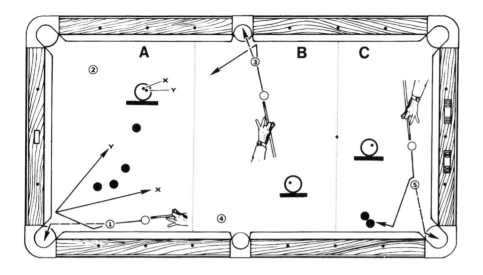

37 Combining follow and English

If you hit the cueball above center and to the right or left of the vertical axis as well, the cueball will be given a rotation that is part topspin and part sidespin. There is no law against it. On the contrary, it is often warmly applauded. Follow affects the path of the cueball as it leaves the ball, English as it leaves the rail. Here are three common shots that illustrate the uses of combined follow and English:

Shot A: The problem is to pocket the 1 and leave the cueball in good shape for the 2. Follow alone will send the cueball to the vicinity of X, behind the interfering balls. A touch of right English, though, as well as follow will make the cueball spurt to the right when it hits the end rail and send it to the vicinity of Y, from which point a sleepwalker could make the 2.

Shot B: How can the 3 be made, and then the 4? By using high left. The high forces the cueball forward to the rail; the left makes it jump to the left to a spot from which the 4 can be cut in the side.

Shot C: The object here is to pocket the 5 and break up the cluster for future use. High right will do the job.

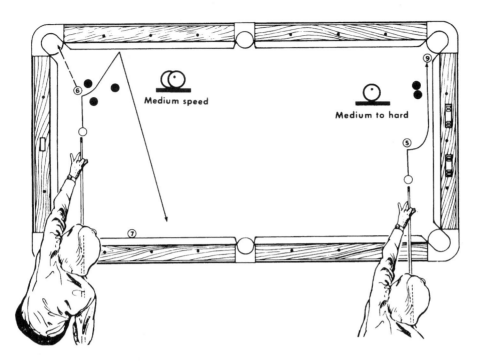

Medium speed

Medium to hard

38 Two advanced follow shots

At the left, the black balls seem to make it impossible to pocket the 6 and get position on the 7. High left English and a medium stroke will force the cueball to follow the curved path as shown. On this particular shot, left English is used as well as follow to keep the cueball away from a possible scratch in the side and to kill the speed off the first rail.

At the right side of the diagram is a position in a nine-ball game. A hard stroke with high follow gives the shooter a chance to end the game in spectacular fashion. When you try this yourself, remember to shoot hard and hit the object ball just a hair to the right of dead center. Still having trouble? Then see the shot executed on *Byrne's Standard Video of Pool, Vol. II.*

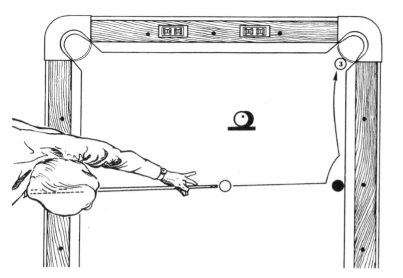

39 Force follow back to the rail

This shot is not easy. Fortunately, it comes up only once in every 176,453 shots. To get the desired spectacular distortion, hit the cueball crisply and very high and hit as much of the black ball as possible without getting a double-kiss. It's much more difficult if the black ball is an inch or two off the rail.

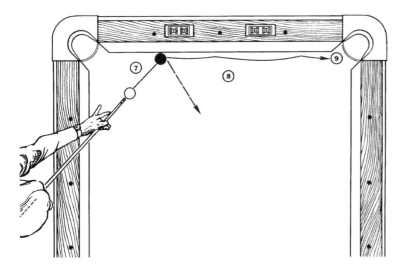

40 Force follow along the rail

By using high follow it is possible to make the cueball go through the black and hug the rail until it pockets the 9. Topspin action of this sort is common in three-cushion billiards, where it is called force-follow double-the-rail. Jacob "The Wizard" Schaefer used to call it "the smash-in shot," according to Thatcher's *Championship Billiards Old and New* (Rand McNally & Co., New York, 1898). It's easier if the cueball approaches the black from a shallower angle.

Note that the dashed line representing the path of the black is drawn from the edge of the ball—that's because the black ball will sink into the rail before it rebounds, a nuance we will confront in Diagram 100 in Section 8.

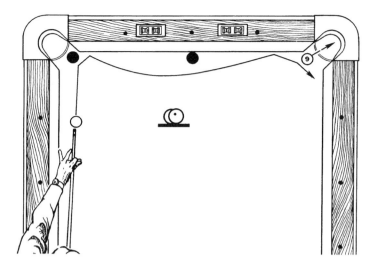

41 Another advanced follow shot

When the object ball is within an inch of the rail, it is possible for even inexperienced players to put a really bizarre bend on the cueball with extreme high English. The shot diagrammed is a favorite of exhibition players wishing to evoke gasps from onlookers. The shot can be made with straight high follow, but I find hitting the cueball a little left of center improves the curving action. Good players with practice can make the cueball bounce a foot or more away from the rail before curving back; that's enough to clear a triangle or line of six or eight balls.

Reference: Many attractive trick shots depend on the ability to make a cueball curve like this. For example, check out the Easy-Action Four-ball Shot in Section 12 of *Byrne's Treasury of Trick Shots.*

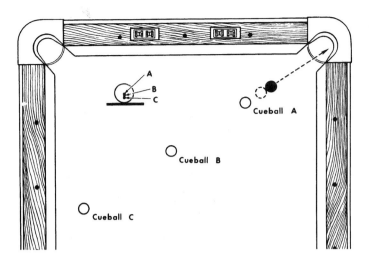

42 An essential weapon: the stop shot

In a straight-in shot, if the cueball *slides* into the object ball without backspin or forward roll, it will stop dead in its tracks. The ability to execute stop shots with assurance is vital to advanced pool playing. Consider the position of the object ball and the three cueballs in the diagram. The goal is to pocket the black ball and leave the cueball in the exact position it was at the moment of impact, as shown by the dashed ball. From position A a centerball hit suffices, providing you don't shoot too softly. From B the cueball has to be hit slightly below center. Position C requires a still lower hit. A centerball hit will also work from B and C if a hard stroke is used; the point is that the cueball has to slide rather than roll into the object ball. When practicing the shot, try to make the cueball stop absolutely dead, not spinning in place or drifting even slightly off line. Note that the harder you hit it the less draw is required.

Reference: Stop-shot capability at all distances is an essential skill. For more, see *Byrne's Standard Video of Pool, Vol. I,* and *Power Pool Workout, Vol. V.*

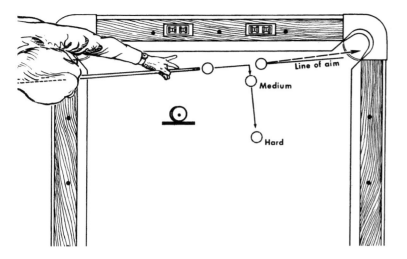

43 The deadball or "stun" shot

A powerful weapon in position play is the deadball shot, which is nothing more than the stop shot at an angle. If you use stop-shot cuing and speed when the object ball is not straight in, the cueball will drift slowly along the right-angle line. The diagrammed shot requires an object ball hit a hair to the right of center. Strike the cueball crisply in the center and what happens? The object ball rockets into the corner pocket and the cueball rolls slowly to the right along the indicated line. Where it stops depends on how hard it was hit. If the cueball rolls to the right or left of the right-angle line it means that there was a slight amount of follow or draw spin on it at the moment of impact—which often is the player's intention. It takes a certain "feel."

In the diagram, if the object ball were an inch or two to the right (as the player looks at the shot), it would be possible to send the cueball the length of the table along the right-angle line (sometimes called the tangent line). British snooker experts have a descriptive term for this play: they call it the "stun" shot.

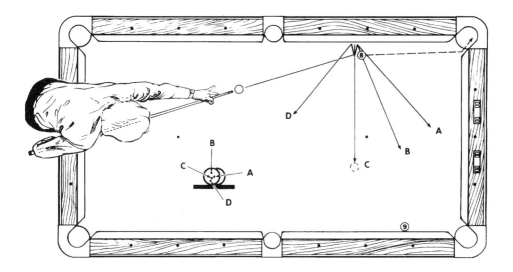

44 One way to use a deadball shot

Say you are faced with this position. What's the best way to pocket the 8-ball and get position on the 9-ball? A, which requires allowance for curve, and B aren't very promising. D is not bad, though the resulting shot is longer than it need be. Best is the stop stroke, or deadball shot, which from this distance would require hitting the cueball slightly below center. The cueball will carom off the side rail and roll slowly to the vicinity of the dashed ball. Both C and D have to be hit harder than A and B because there must be enough backspin supplied initially to overcome the friction of the cloth as the cueball slides toward the 8-ball. In shot D there is still some backspin left at the moment of impact.

draw shots, the use of speed, and the margin of error

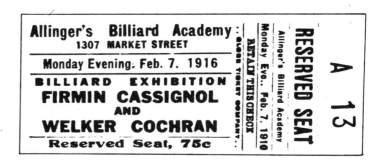

(Byrne Collection)

Secrets of the draw shot

The ability to make a cueball spurt backward off an object ball is something fervently to be desired, for the draw shot is the soul of pool. Without it the game is diminished to the level of, say, bowling. Unfortunately, it's a hard shot for most beginners to learn. Many earnest strivers, for lack of knowledge, spend years without finding the handle.

To draw the ball *with consistency and control,* you must have a properly groomed and chalked tip, a reasonably straight stroke, a snug grip with the left hand so the cue can't stray off course, a hit on the cueball far enough below center to suit the circumstances, and speed appropriate to the distance. Many beginners balk at hitting the cueball more than a little below center, apparently fearing the titters that follow a cueball bouncing absurdly down the table. If your cueball refuses to draw like other people's, try hitting the ball lower than you ever dreamed possible; you won't miscue if your tip is chalked and your bridge is solid.

There are other secrets that the beginner must absorb and make part of his personality. Keep the cue as level as possible. To hit the cueball low, lower the left-hand support and don't raise the butt of the cue. The reasons for this rule are to keep the cueball from curving or bouncing, as it is wont to do when struck from above, and to permit a free follow-through, which is impossible when striking downward. There are exceptions. You must elevate the butt of the cue when trying to draw off a rail or over a ball. The key in such awkward positions is to make sure the extended axis of the cue passes beneath and behind the cueball's center of gravity (which is where the pit would be if the ball were a peach).

Don't omit the follow-through. Many beginners, and a few mistaken experts, think that the cue must be snapped backward after contacting the cueball. Of course for straight-in shots with the cueball close to the object ball you must get the cue out of the way in a hurry to avoid interference with the returning cueball. Nevertheless, whenever possible, you should use a smooth, straight follow-through.

If you find it hard to overcome a natural reluctance to follow through on draw shots, try imagining the cueball several inches beyond its actual position.

NOTE: The diagrams in this book are drawn with the assumption that the cueball weighs the same as the object balls. On most coin-operated tables, the ball-return apparatus depends on the cueball being heavier than the object balls. The disparity makes draw more difficult and follow easier, and distorts the cueball paths on cut shots.

Draw shots are difficult enough without the additional burden of heavy cue-balls. Unable to impart lively draw action and not realizing that the problem lies with their cueballs, hundreds of thousands of tavern players are being denied one of life's sweetest pleasures. In some cases they impute their failures to personal inferiority, and, surrounded as they are by booze, they drink more than they should, which only exacerbates the problem of low self-esteem. Meanwhile, the government remains indifferent. The public drinkers of this country have a serious grievance that is not being redressed. Violence looms, though nothing I say here should be construed as advocating it.

If I were benevolent dictator of the United States, I would make use of a heavy cueball a felony. Every coin-op table in the land would be equipped with three cueballs. The first two scratches would be punished according to normal rules. Whoever scratches with the third and last cueball loses the game. (Note to the makers of coin-op tables and balls: there is no charge for this advice.)

NOTE: How to get lively draw action is explained in detail in *Byrne's Standard Video of Pool, Vol. I.*

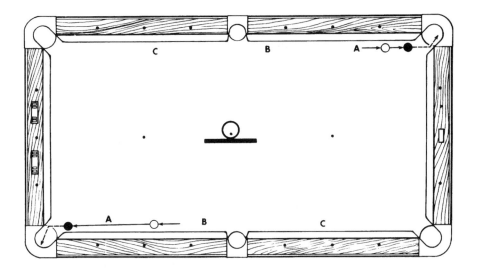

45 Getting the hang of the draw shot

Place the cueball and an object ball about six inches apart as shown in the upper right corner of the diagram. Practice pocketing the black ball and drawing the cueball back to the vicinity of A. If you have trouble, review these fundamentals: Chalk the tip thoroughly, keep the cue level, hold the cue snugly with the left hand, hit the ball crisply and well below center, follow through.

When the balls are close together it is not difficult to draw the cueball to A or even to B. Drawing it five or six feet to C is harder, but within the reach of the average player. The position at the bottom of the diagram is less favorable because the cueball is two diamonds away from the black ball. A harder stroke is required, or a lower hit on the cueball, because the friction of the cloth has more time to work at removing the cueball's backspin. Drawing back to A is not too hard; reaching B and C takes very good execution. An expert player could put the cueball at C to begin with and draw the cueball all the way back to within a foot or two of the starting point, but not every time. Where the cueball will end up on long draw shots can't be predicted with precision. The extent of cueball travel in follow shots is much easier to gauge.

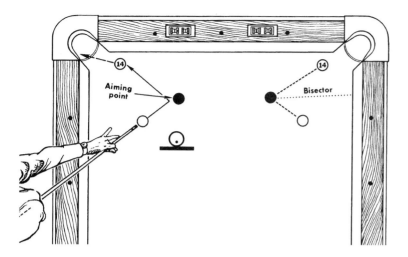

46 Calculating the angle of return

Most good players use judgment when shooting draw-carom shots, but if you have no judgment, there is a geometrical method developed by old-time billiard players you can use. Bisect the angle formed by the three balls (above, right). Where the bisector intersects the rim of the first object ball is the point at which you aim (above, left). How much speed and draw to use can be learned only through practice.

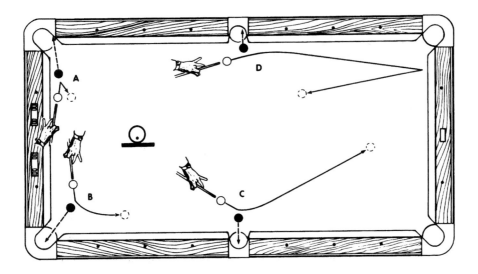

47 Four draw shots at an angle

These four shots illustrate what happens when you use draw at an angle. Each is stroked with the same soft speed and the same low hit on the cueball. The dashed balls indicate roughly where the cueball will come to rest. Note that the thinner the hit, the farther the cueball goes. Just as in follow shots, the cueball moves along the right-angle line before the spin takes effect, which is not visible to the naked eye in a nearly straight-in shot like A.

In shot D, the cueball would likely scratch in the corner pocket if draw were not used; sidespin as well as draw would change the rebound angle off the end rail.

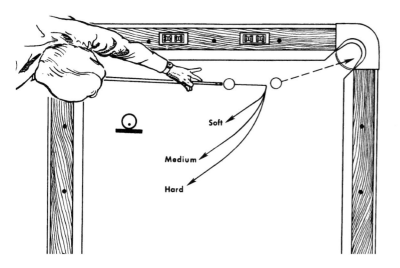

48 How speed affects draw

The harder you hit a draw shot, the farther the cueball travels along the right-angle line before the backspin takes effect. Don't pay too much attention to the exact location of the paths in the diagram, for they will vary depending on the distance between the balls, the speed, the amount of draw, the condition of the cloth, and other factors not worth mentioning. The arrowheads here are not meant to indicate where the cueball will stop, only the direction it will take.

Students trying to learn draw, follow, and stun by studying Volumes I and II of my six-tape video series should be told that the cloth I was using was Simonis 300, which is extremely "fast." Because the coefficient of friction is so low on a napless cloth like that, the curves are wider and broader and easier to see, and the ball rolls and rolls and rolls before stopping. Drawing the cueball is easier because less of the backspin wears off while the cueball is on its way to the object ball.

Reference: See the note below Diagram 21.

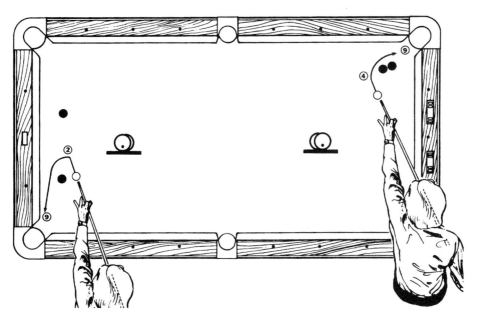

49 Two beautiful draw shots

While draw is usually applied to gain good position for the next shot, it can sometimes be used to pocket a ball on a carom. The two 9-ball shots here aren't easy,
but they aren't impossible either. A tournament player probably wouldn't try them
and neither would a hustler trying to hide his skill. If you want to take a crack at
them even though you aren't ready, put the cueball within six inches of the object
ball and hit the cueball extremely low. Don't shoot too hard. While the cueball
curves whenever you apply backspin on a cut shot, opportunities for making a ball
in this way seldom arise in practical play. Make a draw-curve carom in a serious
game and you'll glow for hours.

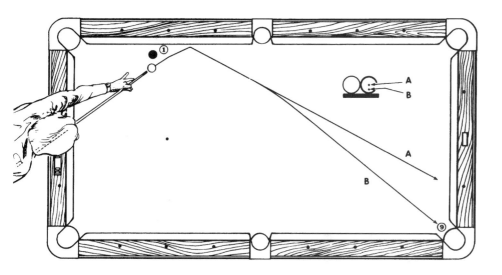

50 Draw action off a rail

Diagram 41 near the end of the last section shows what happens when a topspinning cueball hits an object ball full that is close to a rail. Most of the speed is taken off the cueball but hardly any of the spin, with the result that the cueball path bends back toward the rail. An allied phenomenon takes place when you hit an object ball thin with backspin—the path will bend *away* from the rail, as shown here. Diagrammed is a position from a game of nine-ball. Hitting the 1 extremely thin ("feathering" it) without spin causes the cueball to follow path A. Backspin makes the cueball path undergo a kind of midcourse correction, bending it to conform to line B. The secret lies in hitting the 1 extremely thin and using extremely low draw.

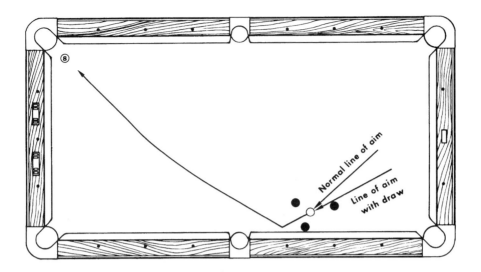

51 Another use of draw off a rail

What would you do here if the 8-ball was the ball you had to hit first? The normal line of aim for a one-rail bank is blocked. A good choice is the one-rail bank with draw, making use of the curve, which you now know will be there if you hit the cueball low. Positions like this come up all the time in games like nine-ball and rotation, in which only the lowest-numbered ball can be contacted first.

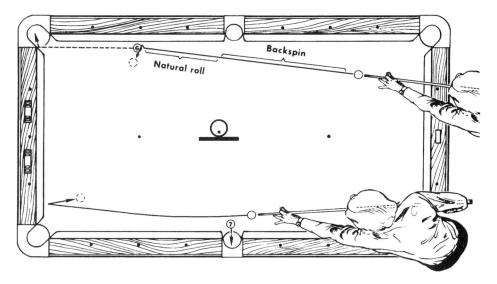

52 How to kill cueball speed with draw

Consider the shot at the top of the diagram. The problem is to make the 6-ball and for reasons of position keep the cueball as close as possible to the rail. One solution would be to shoot very softly. The trouble with that is the cueball will roll off line if the table isn't level or if there are chalk fragments in its path. Most professional players would use the "draw drag" or "skid" shot here. By hitting the cueball below center, more speed can be used because the backspin slows the cueball down as it travels toward the object ball. By the time the 6-ball is reached, the speed is what it would have been if a very soft stroke has been used to begin with, yet no risk of roll-off has been taken. When practicing the shot for the first time, use a striped ball instead of a cueball to make the backspin and skid easier to see. Avoid even the slightest hint of English.

(A reminder on the use of terms. By "English" I mean sidespin; by "follow" topspin; and by "draw" backspin.)

At the bottom of the diagram is a subtle use of draw not often seen—killing cueball speed *after* hitting the object ball. Here the player is faced with a thin cut of the 7-ball into the side pocket. For reasons of position let us assume that forward roll on the cueball must be minimized—that is, the cueball must come to rest as close to the end rail as possible. By using draw, the cueball can be hit firmly enough to pocket the 7 with authority, yet without sending the cueball off the end rail and back to the center of the table. Note that the cueball path bends slightly as the backspin reduces the speed.

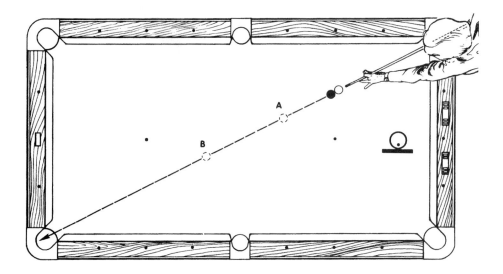

53 The "skid-stop" frozen push shot

Don't give up if you are frozen to an object ball that is aimed directly at a pocket. Shoot straight into the ball without the slightest trace of English but with plenty of draw. The backspin will make the cueball skid to a sudden stop before it follows the object ball into the pocket. How far the cueball goes before stopping depends on how low and how hard you hit it. Softly and very low will halt it at A; a medium stroke will send it to B. Elevate the cue and you can make the cueball stop within inches or even back up.

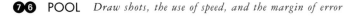

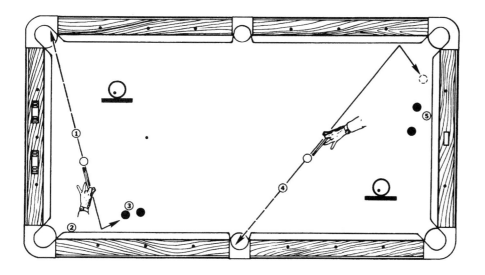

54 Combining draw and English

If the cueball is to be drawn off an object ball into a rail, there may be a reason to hit it on the side as well as below center, that is, to use a combination of backspin and sidespin. Two reasons are diagrammed above. At the left, the player earnestly wishes to make the 1, 2, and 3 in numerical order. Unhappily, the 3 can't be made from its present position. So! Use low left English. The low pulls the cueball back to the rail, the left makes it rebound into the black ball, bumping the 3 into the clear. Unless something terribly unfair happens, the 2 can be made and position played on the 3.

Later in the same game, the player might find himself confronted with the delicate position at the right. A long draw must be made off the 4 to get the cueball into a restricted area from which the 5 can be pocketed. To make sure the cueball draws back far enough but not too far, hit it left of center as well as below center. Now you can use plenty of backspin without fear of overdoing it because when the cueball touches the side rail the "wrong-way" or "hold-up" English will kill the speed.

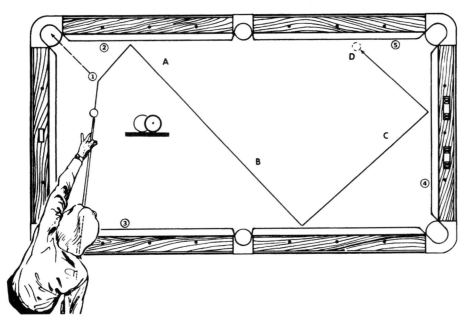

55 Playing position with speed only

Having said so much about the uses of follow, draw, and English, I must empha-
size that a large percentage of shots can be played with none of the above. Centerball hits suffice. Good position on the next ball can often be gained by control
of speed only. In the diagram, cutting the 1-ball into the corner with a very soft
stroke will leave the cueball in the vicinity of A, in good shape for the 2. A little
more speed will carry it to B, in position for the 3. Still more speed is needed to
reach C and a good shot at the 4. D is good for the 5. In each case the hit on the
1 and the English are the same—speed is the only variable. It takes practice and
talent to make the cueball stop within inches of a desired spot on a pattern like
this, but uncanny precision is usually not required.

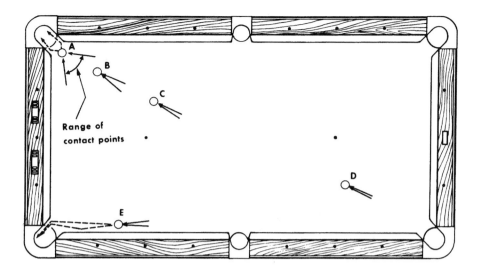

56 The margin of error

Everybody knows that the closer the object ball is to the pocket the easier it is to make, but beginners don't usually grasp the full implications. To play pool expertly it is not enough to simply drive the object ball into a pocket, you often must drive it into a certain *part* of the pocket. That's easy when the ball is "hanging on the lip," not so easy from half the length of the table. The diagram shows how the margin of error shrinks with the length of the shot. The ball at position A can be made by hitting contact points that form an arc of almost 90 degrees, depending on whether the ball is sent into the far right or far left sides of the pocket. Note how quickly the margin of error diminishes for balls at B and C. Even at D there is some leeway, but only a madman would try to exploit it. A ball near a rail, E, has a slightly larger margin of error than appears at first because the ball will drop even if it touches the side rail first.

The margin of error that exists on almost every shot presents the position player with what can be thought of as a margin of freedom. Directing a ball into one part of the pocket or another is called "using the pocket," "cheating the pocket," and "fudging."

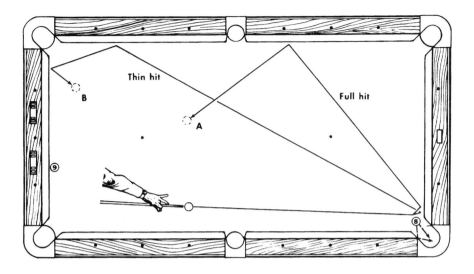

57 Using the margin of error

The problem is to make the 8 in the corner and "get shape," as we say in the pool-hall subculture, on the 9. A very thin hit on the 8 without English sends the cueball to the vicinity of B, a perfect spot for the 9. A fuller hit with the same speed sends the cueball to A, a rotten spot for the 9. The diagram is intended to remind the reader that just because it is easy to pocket the ball doesn't mean he can relax . . . quite the contrary. It is especially embarrassing to fail to get excellent position when the ball is easy to make.

Reference: For more on the subjects mentioned in this section, see Volumes I, II, and V of my videotape series.

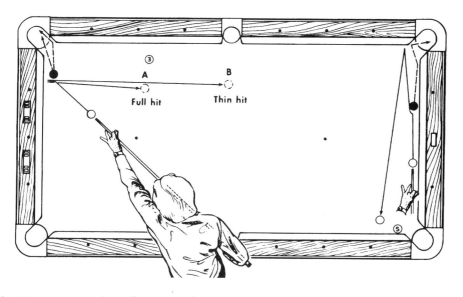

58 More margin of error shots

The thinner you hit the object ball, the less speed is taken off the cueball. At the left above, the player is attempting to cut the black ball into the corner and leave himself a good shot at the 3 in the same corner. A very thin hit, cutting the black ball into the far right side of the pocket, will send the cueball to B, which is fine. A fuller hit on the black with the same speed sends it into the center of the pocket but leaves the cueball short of the desired area.

On the right side of the diagram the player is looking at a straight-in shot and has the problem of getting the cueball to a place from which he can make the 5. Follow might send the cueball after the black into the right corner pocket. Hitting the object ball a hair to the left, however, permitting it to touch the rail before reaching the pocket, creates enough angle for follow to send the cueball along the indicated path. Draw could be used for a similar result, but it is generally easier to estimate the length of a follow than a draw shot, especially when the balls are more than a foot or two apart.

On almost every shot the player has a degree of freedom in his choice of English, speed, and hit. Knowing how to manage the three variables, being able to judge accurately how a change in one affects the others—that's where the artistry of the game lies. Precision in cueball control is the goal toward which to strive. Simply pocketing the object ball is not enough; lots of clowns can do that.

6 throw shots

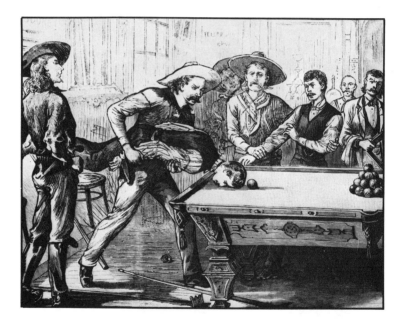

A thinking-man's game, even in Wyoming.
(*Illustrated Police News*, 1887)

Welcome to a weird world

A throw shot is one in which an object ball is forced off line, that is, made to follow a path other than the one suggested by the contact point and the line of centers. There are three situations you will face as a player: when the cueball is separated from the object ball, when the cueball is touching or nearly touching the object ball (see photo below), and when two object balls are touching or nearly touching. They will be explained in that order.

If you are unaware of or unclear about the throw phenomenon, the next few pages are going to improve your game immediately. You will learn why you sometimes miss combinations that you think are "dead" and you will learn how to make others that seem impossible.

A lovely feature of throw shots is that the correct approach doesn't make sense at first blush. It strikes the newcomer as the opposite of what should be done.

The following explanation of throw shots is the most complete ever to appear in print. Certain hustlers are going to hate me for spilling the beans.

Reference: Throw shots are explained with the aid of three cameras on *Byrne's Standard Video of Pool, Vol. I.* See also The Throw Effect on Cut Shots in *Byrne's Advanced Technique.*

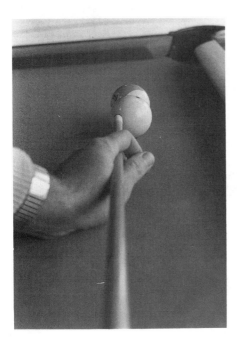

The cueball and the object ball are aimed well to the left of the corner, yet the shot can be made if the balls are touching. Aim straight ahead, use heavy left sidespin, and watch as the object ball is thrown to the right and into the hole.

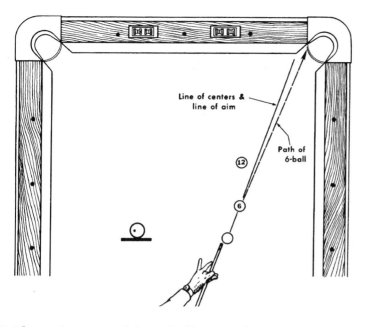

Line of centers &
line of aim

Path of
6-ball

59 Throwing an object ball at a distance

Because there is friction between the balls, a cueball with left-hand spin will grip
the object ball for an instant and throw it off line to the right. In Diagram 25, where
right English is used, there is more to consider than curve and squirt; there is also
the tendency for the object ball to be thrown to the right. Good players sometimes
make use of the way cueball sidespin influences the path of the object ball.

Consider the diagram. The game is straight pool, in which the last ball on
the table is left in place while the rest are racked. The player will have an adequate
break shot if he can pocket the 6-ball and keep the cueball from drifting to the
left, as a straight-in shot on the 12-ball would be useless. Instead of cutting the
6, the expert would hit it head on with a stop-shot stroke and extreme left English, relying on throw to send the 6 enough to the right to enter the pocket. The
cueball will stick in place or move only a hair to the left. Here the throw can be
attributed entirely to the action of English on the object ball because there is not
enough distance between the balls for the cueball to curve.

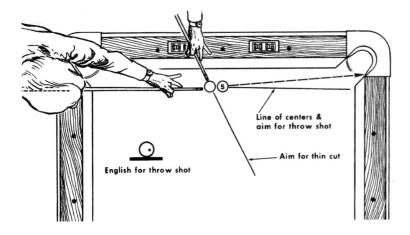

Line of centers &
aim for throw shot

Aim for thin cut

English for throw shot

60 Throwing an object ball up close

Here the cueball is a quarter-inch away from the 5-ball. A line connecting the centers of the two balls intersects the rail an inch away from the point of the corner pocket. Two ways of making the shot are shown. One is to cut the 5 very thin, hitting the cueball very hard in order to transfer enough speed to the 5. The other way is to aim straight at the 5 using right English and shooting softly. Which shot to select depends on where you want the cueball to go. Practice the shot, varying the distance between the balls and the amount of English. Notice how much more you can throw the 5 when the space between the balls is a quarter-inch or less. The trouble with shots involving a gap that small is that it is hard to stop the cue tip before it hits the cueball a second time, which is a foul.

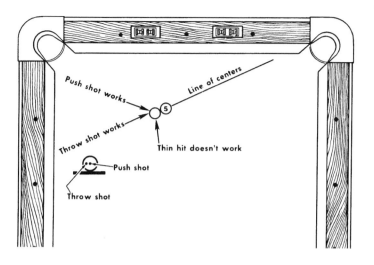

61 Throw shots with a frozen cueball

Now the cueball is frozen to the 5 and the balls are aimed at a point on the rail to left of the corner pocket. With the balls touching, you don't have the option of a thin hit—try it and you'll make matters worse, that is, you'll hit the rail even farther to the left than the line of centers indicates. The straight-ahead throw shot with English works just as well or better when the balls are frozen because you don't have to worry about a double-hit foul. This time, of course, left English is needed. Use a smooth, soft stroke and follow through normally.

With the balls frozen or within a small fraction of an inch of each other there is another option: the push shot, or throwing the object ball with direction rather than English. Use no English and aim your cue at about a 45-degree angle to the line of centers as shown in the diagram. This is the "wrong-way" shot that confounds the newcomer, who instinctively feels that the cueball should be addressed as if a thin cut were being attempted. But the ball is not being cut, it is being pushed. Shoot softly and smoothly, follow through, and watch the 5 mysteriously head for the pocket instead of the rail.

NOTE: The balls don't have to be frozen for the push shot to be an option, but they have to be quite close together, say within a quarter-inch. If the balls are not quite frozen in the above and previous diagrams, the shots could be made three ways: by throwing with English, by pushing without English, and by cutting with an extremely thin hit and a hard stroke.

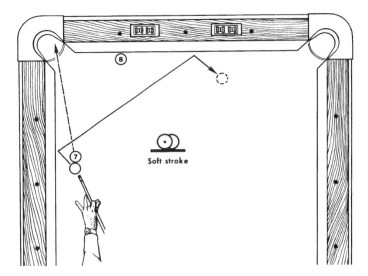

Soft stroke

62 Using the push shot

Say you are stuck to the 7-ball as shown. With proper technique you can not only make the 7 but get perfect position on the 8. Some fairly good players would butcher this shot. The correct way is to push the 7 into the pocket rather than throwing it in with English. By using the push (or directional throw) shot, the cueball travels to a good place for the 8. Remember that when the cueball is frozen or very close to the object ball, the object ball can be thrown off line with either English (straight-ahead hit) or direction (no English, angled hit). Pick one or the other depending on which best satisfies positional needs.

The student will have to experiment to get a feel for the limits involved. Forty-five degrees appears to be the angle that produces the maximum throw on push shots when the cueball is frozen to the object ball, using a centerball hit. What is the maximum possible throw? About a foot over the length of the table, using a combination of directional throw and English throw.

To eliminate throw without shooting straight at the ball to which the cueball is frozen, use an aiming angle of close to 90 degrees—that is, shoot almost straight across the line of centers so that only a small percentage of the cueball's speed is transferred to the object ball.

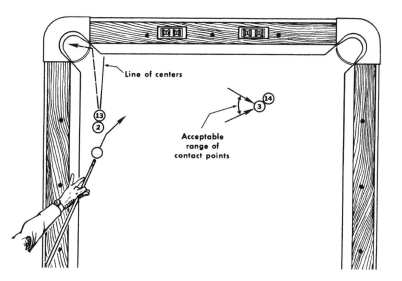

Line of centers

Acceptable
range of
contact points

63 How to throw frozen object balls

For those who don't already possess it, the information in this diagram is priceless, or is at least worth the cost of this book, whichever is smaller. At the left, the 2 and the 13 are lined up to hit the rail on the right side of the pocket. To make the 13 the 2 must be hit on the right side. Children, musicians, and foreigners always seem to want to hit it on the left, as if the 13 could be *cut* into the pocket. When the balls are frozen, the ball must be hit on what seems to be the wrong side. The cueball spin is immaterial, giving the player great freedom in positioning the cueball for the next shot. (Cueball spin can't be transmitted beyond the first ball.)

At the right, the 3 and the 14 are aimed a little to the left of the pocket. The 14 can be thrown into the pocket if the 3 is hit almost anywhere on the left side. Don't hit the 3 *too* thin, though, or the 14 will never reach the pocket.

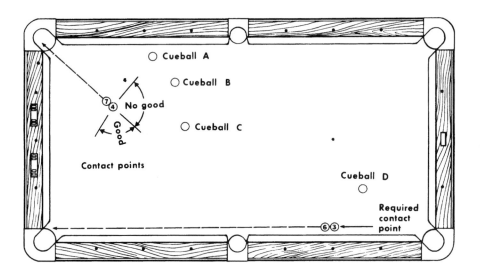

64 Why "dead" combinations are missed

Players who cry "I thought it was dead!" after missing apparently cinch combinations usually don't fully understand how frozen balls are thrown. Take the 4-7 in this position. They are frozen and lined up with the left side of the pocket. Because there is a sizable margin of error for balls this close to a pocket, the 4 can be struck head-on or anywhere on the left side. However, if the 4 is struck to the right of the line of centers, the area labeled "No good," the 7 will be thrown to the left and won't go in. Thus the shot is impossible with cueball A. It can be made with cueball B if the 4 is cut very thin. The shot is easy with cueball C because the left side of the 4 is readily accessible.

The 3-6 combination is lined up so far from the pocket that there is no margin of error to speak of. The only safe place to hit the 3 is the one indicated by the arrow. If cueball D is shot straight into the 3, the 6 will be thrown against the rail before reaching the corner and will not go in.

Cueball C and the 4-7 combination is a case in which you must minimize the throw if you hope to pocket the ball. In a game you might find it impossible to hit the left side of the 4 because of interfering balls. If the 4 can be hit squarely and with a hard stroke, the throw will be minimized and the 7 might go in. Then again, it might not.

Reminder: The balls don't have to be quite frozen.

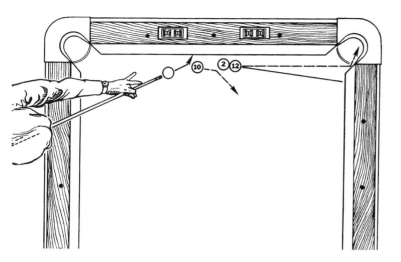

65 The "third-ball" principle

Now that you know how to throw a ball that is quite close or frozen to another, this diagram shouldn't surprise you. The 2-12 pair is aimed at the rail to the right of the pocket. To throw the 12 to the left and into the pocket, the 2 must be struck on the right side, but not necessarily by the cueball. Any "third ball" will do, in this case the 10. Note how the shooter is cutting the 10 into the right side of the 2. Most beginners would miss this shot by driving the 10 too squarely into the 2. Remember that it is where the *third ball* contacts the second ball that determines which way the first ball will be thrown.

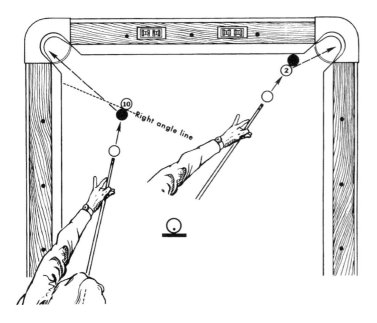

Right angle line

66 How to distort frozen kiss shots

In some positions it is possible to force the object ball in frozen kiss shots to follow a path that crosses or diverges from the right-angle line. Two examples are diagrammed. At the left, the use of extreme draw will transfer a touch of follow to the black ball and cause its path to bend toward and possibly into the pocket.

At the right is an even less promising arrangement. By hitting the 2 squarely, rather hard, and with extreme low, the 2-ball can be made. The black ball will sink into the rail and rebound out of the way. It's no cinch.

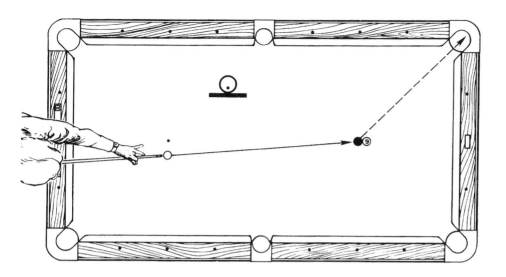

67 The force-through, two-ball spot shot

The most common situation in which force-through action is called for is when the ball you must hit first is on the spot with another ball behind it. In the diagram, the black ball can be propelled directly into the corner pocket, though even the greatest players can't do it more often than half the time. Use draw and hit the black ball full in the face. Try to draw the cueball straight back.

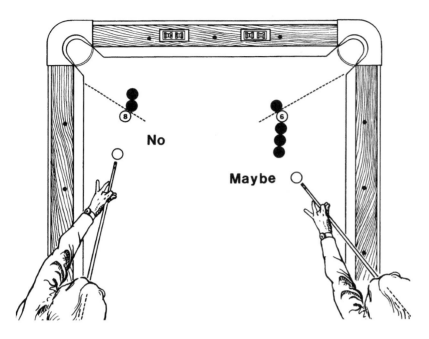

68 Two more "force-through" positions

The 8-ball can't be forced through the black ball it is frozen to because a second ball prevents the first one from getting out of the way in time. The shot as diagrammed is impossible.

At the right, the 6-ball can be forced through the black ball that is restraining it even though it can't be hit squarely by a backspinning cueball. The principle here is that three balls are pushing the 6 and only one is holding it back—the result is that the single ball will yield slightly to the greater weight opposed to it, if you want to think of it in those terms, enabling the 6 to cross the right-angle line and go into the pocket.

Remember these two ideas when studying a cluster for a shot that will go.

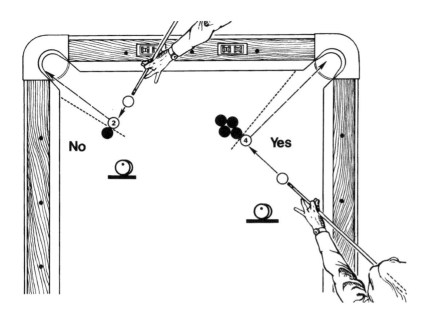

No

Yes

69 The "pull-back" frozen kiss shot

A trace of backspin can be transferred to an object ball by topspin on the cueball, provided the object ball is supported by more than one ball. At the right in the diagram, the 4-ball can be made to "pull back" from the right-angle line by using follow on the cueball. The shot at the left is impossible because the 2-ball isn't solidly enough supported.

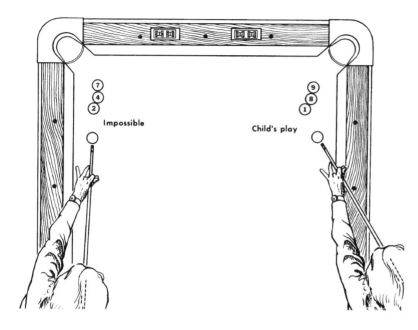

Impossible

Child's play

70 Frozen three-ball combinations

At the left, there is no way the 7-ball can be pocketed by hitting the 2 first, because it is contacting the 4 on the wrong side. The contact point can't be changed no matter how the 2 is hit; the shot is impossible. The shot at the right can hardly be missed because the 1 (the third ball) is touching the 8 on the proper side. It makes no difference where you hit the 1, provided enough force is used to propel the 9 into the pocket. Incidentally, if the cueball at the right were shot across the table into the 4-ball, the 7 would go in because the cueball would be the third ball in relation to the 7 and would impart throw action from the proper side.

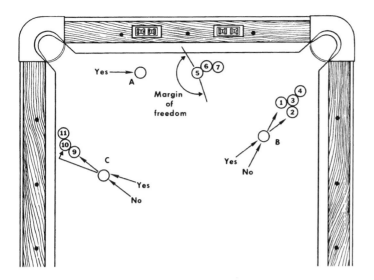

71 More on frozen three-ball combinations

Shot A shows the tremendous leeway enjoyed by the shooter when a three-ball combination is "on." shot B teaches a valuable lesson: Hit the 1-ball anywhere and the 4 won't go, but hit the 2-ball anywhere and it will. Decisions like this are made frequently by players looking for combinations in clusters of balls. In shot C, the 10-ball must be hit on the left to throw the 11 to the right and into the pocket; therefore the 9-ball is anathema. To make the shot, go to the rail first.

The reader will have to discover for himself how the throw effect is altered by slight spaces between the balls, by various third-ball contact points, and by speed. To illustrate every possible arrangement would take a book of infinite bulk and an author of infinite patience, neither of which is imaginable.

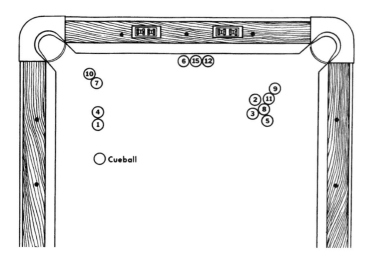

72 Three-ball combinations and beyond

From the cueball position given, is it possible to make the 10 by hitting the 1? The 12 by hitting the 6? The 9 by hitting the 2, 3, or 5? Decide before reading on. The 7-10 combination is aimed to the right of the pocket, which means that the 7 must be hit on the right side. By shooting into the 1, the 4 becomes the third ball. The 4 will hit the 7 on the wrong side, so the shot should be shunned.

The 6-15-12 group is lined up straight into the pocket. Because the 6-ball (the third ball) is already touching the 15 at the right spot, the 6 can be hit almost anywhere and the 12 will go in. If the cueball is shot directly into the 15, the 12 will be thrown against the rail and will rebound away from the pocket.

The 5-ball cluster at the right should present no problem in analysis now that you are among the cognoscenti. The 11 must be hit on the left side to throw the 9 into the pocket; therefore no combination involving the 8 will work. Knock the 2 into the 11 and the 9 will go.

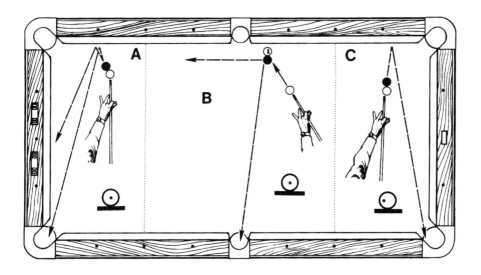

73 Influencing bank shots with throw

Because throw action is so pronounced on banks, shots can be made that at first sight seem impossible. Set up these three examples and ask a friend if they can be made.

Shot A: The balls are aimed at the side rail at an angle that suggests a return to the middle of the end rail. By shooting perpendicularly to the side rail (directional push), the black ball can be banked in the corner. Shooting straight at the black with left English (English throw) won't work here because the cueball will interfere with the black on its way back.

Shot B: Even though the balls are perpendicular to the side rail, the 1-ball will bank across the table at an angle into the side if the black is hit as shown.

Shot C: Here directional push will result in a kiss-out. Use English throw.

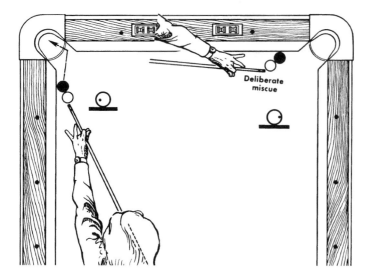

Deliberate miscue

74 Two throw shots—one illegal

Don't worry about the rail on throw shots; pretend it doesn't exist. The black ball at the left in the diagram can be made either with English or direction. At the right the angle is too severe for a legal shot, but an illegal deliberate miscue will do the trick. Aim to hit the cueball at the far right edge. A faster-than-the-eye-can-follow double-kiss will send the black ball into the pocket as slick as a whistle. Don't do it in a game for money, though, if you value your thumbs.

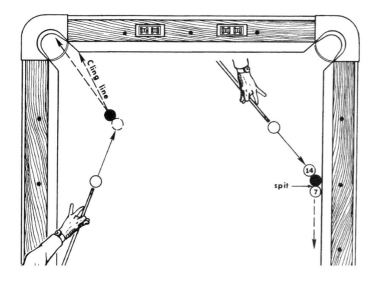

75 The phenomenon of "cling"

Sometimes when trying to cut a ball into a pocket you will notice that the cue-ball seems to stick to it for an instant. Even though the cueball hits the right contact point, the object ball skids for a few inches like an ashtray (Irving Crane's simile) along an improper line instead of going into the pocket with natural roll. I call this excessive throw "cling."

Cling occurs when the normal friction between the ball surfaces is increased by fingerprints, sweat, french-fry grease, hair oil, chalk, and other odious substances. It can occur even if the balls are brand new or newly cleaned; if you chalk your cue and hit the cueball, a smudge of chalk is transferred to the cueball . . . and if that smudge hits the object ball—cling!

While we are on the subject of odious substances, look at the position at the right in the diagram, which is an old trick shot of the challenge variety. You can hit the 14 and run the 7 down the rail into the corner pocket (out of the diagram) every time but the sucker whom you are fleecing can't. And why not? Because while adopting a contemplative pose you manage to stick your forefinger into your mouth. When setting up the balls for your turn, you moisten the contact point, thus greatly reducing the coefficient of friction between the black ball and the 7. Without normal friction the black can't transmit "throw" to the 7 and the 7 will stay on the rail. I once did this twenty times in a row without my highly intelligent but nevertheless hapless dupe uncovering the subterfuge.

Reference: See also When to Cut and When to Throw in *Byrne's Advanced Technique.* To learn how to throw a combination without hitting it on one side or another, see Throw Shots, Tangent Lines, and More in *Byrne's Wonderful World.* The amazing distortions possible by doctoring the contact point (secretly if you enjoy robbing your friends) with chalk, thus raising the friction between balls, are covered in the section called Choice Inner Secrets in *Byrne's Treasury of Trick Shots.* Also see the section on "secret substances" in *Byrne's Standard Video of Trick Shots, Vol. III.*

7

practice methods

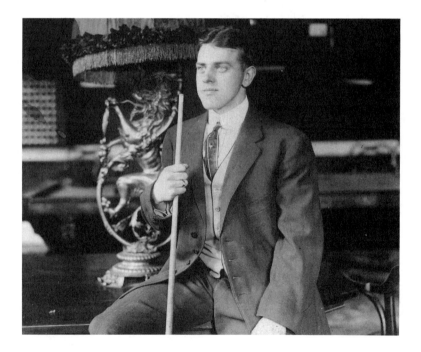

The fabulous Willie Hoppe in 1910 at the age of twenty-three. He won his first world championship in 1906 in Paris and his last in 1952 in San Francisco. It's hard to imagine that anyone ever again—in any sport or game—will win world titles separated by so many years. (Library of Congress)

Getting the most out of practicing

What should you do when you are alone at the table? Breaking the rack apart and pocketing balls at random is fun and is good practice if you don't get careless and sloppy, which results not in improvement but in the reinforcement of bad habits. I tend to agree with those who maintain that pool is best regarded as an amusement rather than as life itself, but I also believe that a thing done well is more amusing than a thing done poorly. So systematize at least part of your practice time. Work on stop shots, draw, follow, English, long shots, speed control, banks, and shooting left-handed (to minimize the need for the awkward mechanical bridge). Try to make the cueball go to certain spots. Bear down. Concentrate. Pretend the county championship is riding on every stroke. Go through this book and try every example.

To force yourself to plan ahead, scatter the fifteen balls around on the table so that no ball is within six inches of another ball or of a rail. Put the cueball anywhere and try to run the table, shooting the balls in any order, without allowing the cueball to touch a rail.

Readers really serious about mastering the game should drop out of school, quit their jobs, and get a divorce.

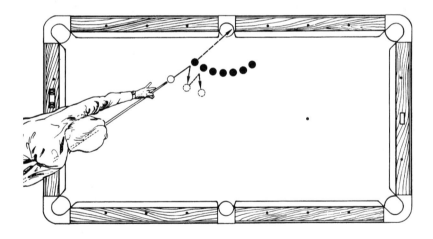

76 A draw-shot drill

Starting from this position, see if you can pocket the balls in order from one end to the other, using draw to gain position. The trick is to use various parts of the pocket depending on the angle of the shot. Beginners should use a row of three or four balls, experts nine or ten.

A game that teaches cueball control

Most players spend far too much of their practice time pocketing balls and not nearly enough on positioning the cueball. Working on shots you usually miss or that are hard to make is OK, but it is more productive to set up easy shots and try to make the cueball bend to your will. A player who thinks ahead and has an obedient cueball doesn't need outstanding shotmaking ability because he usually leaves himself something easy.

To encourage students to practice cueball control, I have devised a game involving the ten shots given in the next seven diagrams. In each case it's easy to pocket the ball. The challenge is to make the cueball behave properly. The shots are worth one point each (perfect score: ten) and the players have two chances at each one. On shots with a "target zone," the cueball must stop entirely within it to score. Don't worry about duplicating the exact paths in the diagrams; the only condition is to get the cueball to the required destination. Also, the exact position of the balls is not critical; players can make minor adjustments before shooting if they like.

If you play alone, keep track of your scores as a measure of progress. As a contest against one or more players, it's best to let each player try one or two shots per turn rather than all ten. Ties can be broken by playing the game again without the second-chance option, or by using shots of your own devising.

The name of the game is Position. If people would play it once in a while instead of the same old eight-ball and nine-ball all the time, America would enjoy a better class of pool player. See the reference note on next page.

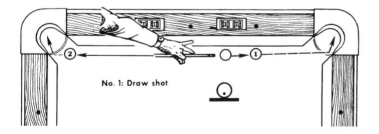

No. 1: Draw shot

77 Position shot 1—precision draw

The 1-ball is one diamond from the corner, the 2-ball is in the jaws, and the cueball is wherever you want it to be. The object is to sink both balls on one shot with draw.

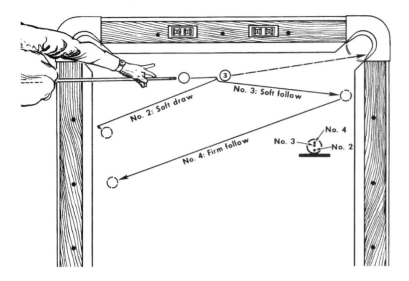

78 Position shots 2, 3, & 4—draw and follow

Place the cueball and 3 approximately as shown. The object of shot 2 is to pocket the 3 and draw the cueball to within one ball-width of the left-hand side rail. Shot 3: Pocket the 3 and by using follow leave the cueball within one ball-width of the right-hand side rail. Shot 4: Pocket the ball and with follow make the cueball bank across the table and stop within two ball-widths of the left side rail.

Reference: All ten position practice shots diagrammed here are demonstrated in *Byrne's Power Pool Workout, Vol. V,* a videotape entirely devoted to practice methods and drills.

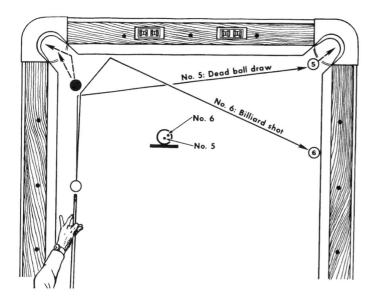

79 Position shots 5 & 6—draw and cushion carom

Shot 5 calls for making the black ball and the 5-ball on one stroke using draw. In shot 6 the cueball must pocket the black ball and rebound off the rail into the 6-ball.

Reference: See also The Best Ways to Practice in *Byrne's Advanced Technique.*

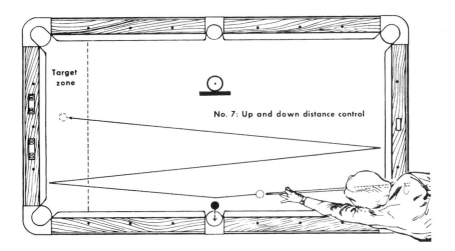

80 Position shot 7—up and down distance control

After a thin cut of the black ball into the side pocket, the cueball must travel up and down the table and come to rest within one diamond of the end rail. (On shots like this the shooter must integrate two variables, speed and thinness of hit. The thinner the hit the less speed is needed. Under game conditions, a third variable, English, must be weighed and blended with the others.)

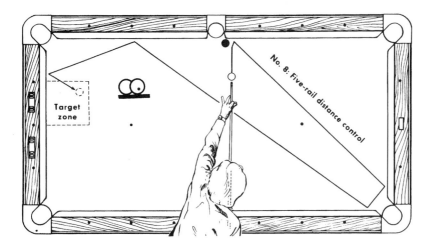

81 Position shot 8—five-rail distance control

The cueball must cut a ball into the side pocket and travel four or five rails to die within a target zone one diamond wide and one diamond deep.

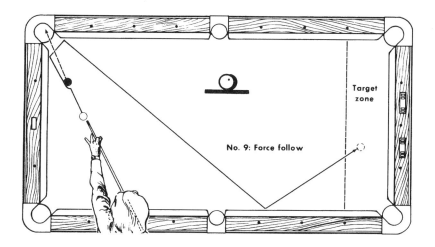

No. 9: Force follow

82 Position shot 9—force follow

This takes a firm stroke and high right-hand English. After pocketing the 9-ball, the cueball follows through three rails into the target zone.

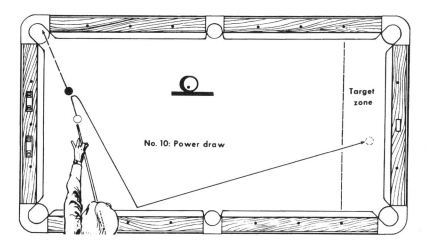

No. 10: Power draw

83 Position shot 10—power draw

The most difficult of the ten position practice shots and far beyond the reach of most beginners. Not only must the cueball be given lively draw action but left-hand English as well so that when it touches the rail it will spurt toward the target zone. Think twice before gambling with anybody who can make this shot consistently. (A restriction: The cueball must touch the side rail on the near side of the side pocket.)

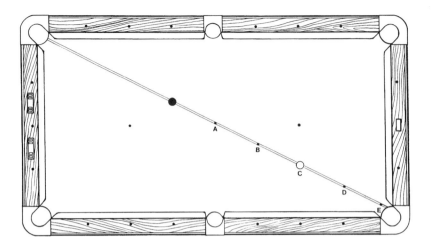

84 Learning the straight-in shot

Miss a cut shot and you can blame it on misjudging the angle or the amount of throw. Miss a shot that is straight and there can be only one thing wrong: your fundamentals. That's why straight-in shots are so important—develop deadly accuracy, and all your other shots will improve as well. Stretch a length of half-inch paper tape, available in the bandage section of any drugstore, diagonally across the table. Mark points opposite the diamonds. The idea is to make a series of progressively longer shots. Position an object ball as shown in the diagram and begin with the cueball at A. The tape guides your eye and your stroke and makes it easy to keep the cue in perfect alignment. If you hit the cueball in the exact center (zero sidespin) and follow straight through so that the tip comes to rest on the tape or directly above it, the shot is almost bound to be successful.

Try it as a progressive exercise and chart your progress. The object ball is always placed as shown. If you miss from B, go back to A. The cueball is always placed one position farther away if you make the shot, one position closer when you miss. The number of shots it takes to be successful from E is the only number you need to record.

NOTE: It's instructive to try a few of the shots with sidespin just to see how much harder they are. Sidespin is treacherous!

Reference: I explain the straight-in drill more fully in the April 1997 issue of *Billiards Digest* magazine and demonstrate it on the videotape *Power Pool Workout.* Valuable are Bob Jewett's articles on progressive drills in *Billiards Digest,* December 1992 and December 1995.

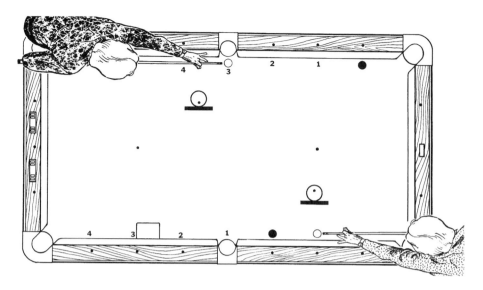

85 Progressive follow and draw

There's nothing like the progressive approach to keep you focused and trying your best, which is the key to rapid improvement. At the top of the diagram is a draw-shot drill. Start with the cueball at position 1. Pocket the black ball and draw back to the starting point or beyond. Replace the black ball and put the cueball at 2 and draw back at least to 1. From 3, draw back at least to 1. When you miss, go back to the next closest position. See where you end up after ten tries. A variation is to see if you can draw back each time to the cueball position or beyond. It's not easy to start at 4, pocket the black ball, and draw back to 4 or beyond, especially on coarse cloth that quickly removes backspin.

At the bottom of the diagram is a systematic follow-shot drill. The starting position is always as shown. The goal is to run the black ball down the rail into the corner pocket and leave the cueball on a sheet or two of typing paper placed successively at 1, 2, 3, and 4. As you improve, use a single sheet, then half a sheet. If you succeed at position 3 (shown), move the paper to 4; if you fail at 3, move it back to 2. Chart your progress in a notebook. If you have a friend who also wants to improve, compete with him or her in progressive drills like these.

Professional singers and musicians practice scales—you think you're so great you don't have to?

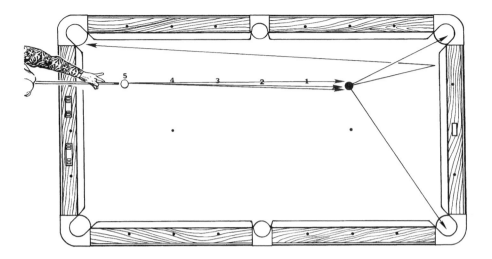

86 Progressive cuts and banks

This setup is designed to help you improve your accuracy on long banks and two kind of cuts. The black object ball is always placed one diamond from the side rail and two from the end rail. The progressive cueball positions are numbered. For easy replacement of the balls, mark the positions with gummed punched-hole re-inforcements, which are perfect for repetitive drills because balls settle quickly in the center hole. Practice all three shots by moving closer when you miss, farther away when you score. Record the finishing position after ten tries.

It's important to place the balls in marked positions so that the practice shots are identical, otherwise keeping records is meaningless.

Now that you know how progressive drills work, make up your own to work on whatever you feel is weakest in your game. Keep records to help you compete against yourself.

Reference: The follow drill, the above three-shot drill, and the line-up drill (next page) are demonstrated on *Power Pool Workout.*

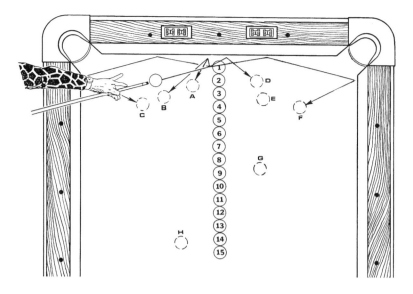

87 The straight-line pick-off drill

There are an infinite number of ways you can arrange fifteen balls on the table to practice shotmaking and cueball control. I like the straight line shown in the diagram because it's from one of my favorite games, line-up straight pool. (See Section 16, Rules of Major Pool Games, at the end of Book One.) In the game, if you succeed in running the table, the balls are replaced in a straight line . . . but not necessarily in the indicated numerical order. Each ball made counts one point and you can make them in any sequence. As a practice drill, start with the balls in a line and the cueball in an ideal position close to the rail. Shots must be called . . . no slop allowed.

Send the end ball into the corner pocket and with slight draw and left spin bring the cueball to A for the 2-ball. Or use a little more draw and spin and bring the cueball to B. Still more draw and the correct speed will send the cueball on a two-rail path to C. Those aren't the only options. A little follow will send the cueball to D, from where a soft draw off the 2-ball will leave you at E for the 3-ball. Or, from the starting position, the cueball can be sent two rails with follow and right sidespin to position F. The choice of paths depends on the angle of the shot.

After picking off four or five balls, it is usually necessary to disturb the line with a follow shot that forces the cueball to burrow through the remaining balls. It's possible to pick off seven balls before breaking the line, but to make the eighth ball you'll need almost perfect position (G), an almost simultaneous hit on the

8-ball and 9-ball, and some left English to help throw the 8-ball into the upper right corner pocket. Occasionally the player loses position when making balls at the start and finds the cueball at the other end of the line. The end ball (the 15) can be made directly into the side if the cueball is at H. Otherwise, a bank shot might be necessary.

In a game of line-up straight pool, you try to run the table and leave the cueball near the rail end of the line to start the sequence again. As a practice drill (assuming you aren't a player that can run the table almost every time from a good starting position), shoot till you miss, jot down the number of balls made, and start over. It's an enjoyable way to develop precision cueball control.

Another good game that lends itself well to charting progress is Equal Offense, also explained in Rules of Major Pool Games.

Reference: For five pages on the great game of line-up straight pool, see the section called The Games People Play in *Byrne's Wonderful World.*

Three "soft-touch" drills

Place fifteen balls on the table in five rows of three, each ball on the intersection of imaginary lines connecting the rail diamonds. Start with the cueball anywhere and try to pocket all fifteen balls without letting any ball touch the back of a pocket. John Delaveau, head referee of the Pro Billiards Tour, recommends this as a way of developing a soft touch.

With the same array, try running the table without letting the cueball touch a rail, a challenge favored by Bob Jewett, who teaches pool teachers. The drills are seen on the *Power Pool Workout* video.

To help beginners develop a soft touch, try a drill suggested by Ed Nagel, veteran Northern California pool teacher. Set up a straight-in shot with the object ball a foot from the pocket and the cueball another foot away. The idea is to pocket the ball in as many strokes as possible, nudging it just an inch or two each time. Five strokes is fair; ten is good.

miscellaneous inside stuff

8

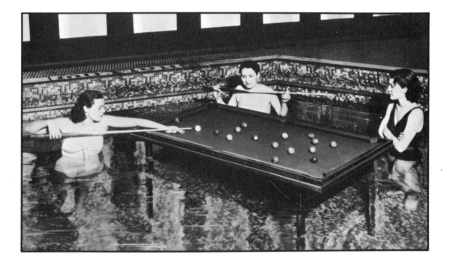

Pool in a pool. Left: Eleanor Holm, swimming sensation of the 1936
Olympics. Center: Georgia Veatch, Midwest Ladies' Pool Champion.
Right: Mrs. Paul Gallico.
(The Billiard Archive)

Audiences frequently marvel at the clever shots that professional players uncork during tournament games. What they don't realize is that the performance is sometimes not as inspired as it seems. The pro may simply be applying one of a large stock of well-known tricks. We'll discuss a few of those tricks in this section along with a number of fundamental ideas that are hard to classify.

Not all tricks, of course, are well known. The interference system described on the next two pages is still pretty much a secret even though it was born decades ago (February 23, 1978, between 7:00 P.M. and midnight).

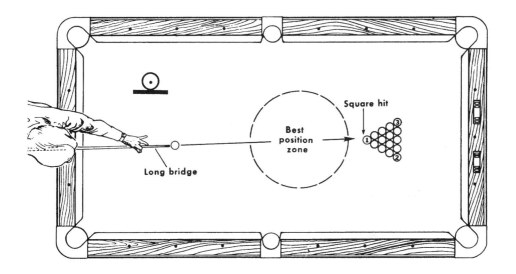

88 The open break

Rotation, eight-ball, nine-ball, and many other pool games begin with an open break, in which the cueball is sent into the racked balls with maximum force. For best results, place the cueball on the head string alongside the head spot (not on or behind the spot, which can act as a ramp to get the cueball airborne), position the left hand farther away from the cueball than usual, grip the cue with the right hand near the rear of the wrapping, and hit the 1-ball as squarely as possible. Try to leave the cueball within the large dashed circle. Scratching on the break is a disaster against a good player, so don't let the cueball run wild by using follow or by hitting the 1-ball on the side.

Reference: See Twenty Keys to a Killer Break in *Byrne's Advanced Technique.*

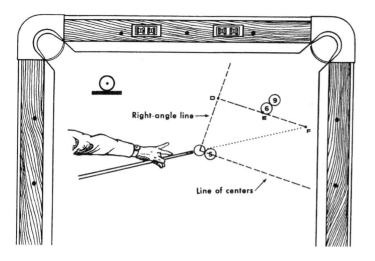

Right-angle line →

Line of centers

89 Jewett's interference system—I

Sometimes the cueball's path to a target is blocked by a ball against which it is frozen. Is there a way to find a line of aim that will send the cueball through the interfering ball and into the target? Many players aim along the bisector of the angle formed by the target, the cueball, and the line of centers of the two frozen balls. That method is no good at all when only a little of the interfering ball is in the way and only fairly good when most of it is. Sick and tired of the imprecision, Bob Jewett worked out a method that works well for every degree of interference. You have to have a knack for geometry to visualize it quickly enough to use in a game.

In the diagram, the shooter would like to find a line of aim that will make the cueball push through the 5-ball and into the 6 at point E to pocket the 9. Here's how to do it. Imagine a line at right angles to the line of centers from the center of the cueball. Imagine a line DE that is perpendicular to the right-angle line. Extend line DE to F so that EF equals DE. F is the aiming point, as indicated by the dotted line.

Use a centerball hit on the cueball, firm speed, and a smooth follow-through stroke.

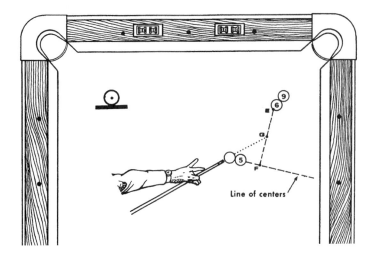

Line of centers

90 Jewett's interference system—II

You may find it easier to apply the Jewett system in the manner diagrammed here. Drop a perpendicular from the target point, E, to the line of centers forming line EF. The midpoint of EF—which is here labeled G—is the aiming point. This method is easier to visualize when most of the 5-ball is interfering. The previous method is best when only a little of the 5-ball is interfering. Both give exactly the same aiming line.

A slight source of error results from the throw effect described in Section 6. To compensate, imagine the line the 5 will take when throw is considered and build the geometry on that line rather than on the true line of centers. The result will be an aiming point that is a hair closer to the target.

Because of the way the interfering ball pushes the cueball to one side, it's possible to miscue slightly on this shot even with a centerball hit. When that happens you'll miss the target point by several inches on the left.

To test the system and get an idea of the slight allowance that must be made for throw, freeze a cueball to another ball and place them both against the end rail *at any point.* Shooting the cueball through the interfering ball toward the center of the side pocket will make it scratch in the far corner. (The Jewett theory in its purest form requires point E in the diagrams to be located at the center of the cueball at the moment of contact. Putting point E at the point of contact as shown helps provide the correction needed to compensate for throw.)

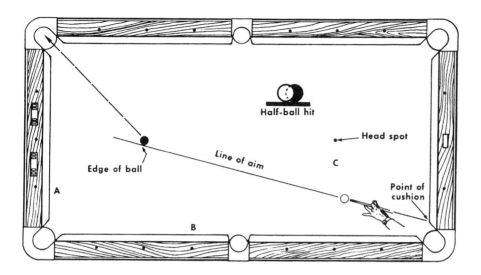

Half-ball hit

Head spot

Line of aim

Edge of ball

C

A

Point of cushion

B

91 A method of making the spot shot

The spot shot comes up over and over and the ability to make it consistently is essential. Two methods have been developed to take some of the guesswork out of it. In *The 99 Critical Shots in Pool* (Quadrangle, New York, 1977), former national champion Ray Martin recommends placing the cueball half a diamond from the head spot (at C in the diagram) and shooting the cueball at the center of the end rail, paying no attention to the object ball. A better method, in my opinion, is the one advocated by 1975 intercollegiate champion Bob Jewett, which involves a half-ball hit. A half-ball hit is easy to make because all you have to do is direct the center of the cueball at the edge of the object ball. Place the cueball on a line running from the left edge of the object ball to the point of the cushion at the corner pocket, as diagrammed. If the cueball is struck lightly above center with moderate speed, it will knock the spotted ball into the pocket, carom to the end rail at A and to the side rail at B. (See Diagram 11 in Book Two for more on the half-ball hit.)

Jewett, incidentally, now a research scientist for Hewlett-Packard in California, is the world's foremost authority on the physics governing the behavior of colliding spheres on green cloth.

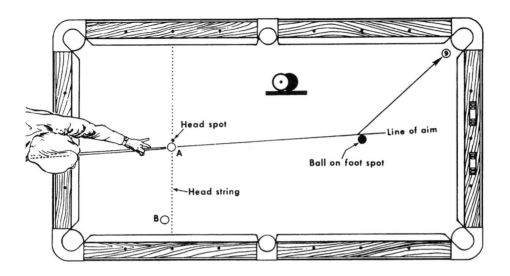

Head spot

Line of aim

A

Ball on foot spot

Head string

B

92 The carom spot shot

It's hard to name an American who hasn't been faced with this: The cueball can be placed anywhere behind the head string, the ball that must be hit first is on the foot spot, and a ball that would be nice to make is hanging in the jaws of the corner pocket. Assume that the diagram is the final scene from a game of nine-ball, with the 8 on the spot and the 9 on the brink. Most players would put the cueball near B and try to drive the 8 into the 9. Easier is the carom from A using soft speed and a half-ball hit. (Soft speed is needed here to avoid following the 9-ball into the pocket.) To convince yourself that the carom is better—and not just because you won't leave a combination if you miss—put the 9-ball on the rail just outside the jaws, relocate the cueball slightly, and try both shots ten times.

Reference: See The Importance of the Half-ball Hit as well as How to Aim Carom Shots in *Byrne's Advanced Technique.*

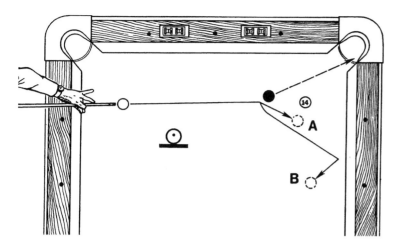

93 The soft versus the firm option

To pocket the black ball and get shape on the 14, should you baby the ball to land at A, or use more speed to land at B? Almost all top players would take the latter course. The first is too precious and cozy—the black ball might not reach the pocket, or one of the balls might be deflected by a crumb of chalk or drift off course by reason of the table's or its own lopsidedness. Going for B enables the shooter to use a more authoritative and confident stroke; with extra speed, crumbs and roll-offs are less a factor. Sometimes, of course, the path to B is blocked and you must trust the equipment and your own soft touch.

Although unrelated to the main point of the diagram, there is an additional disadvantage to A. To make the 14 from there would require the use of the wooden bridge. No sense saddling yourself with that when you can avoid it.

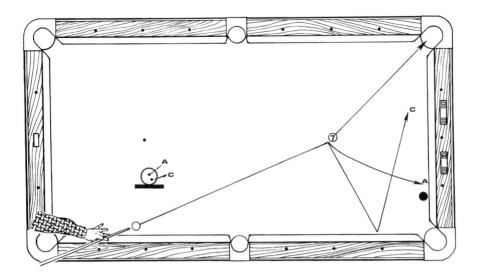

94 Another choice between soft and firm

Let's say the cueball is behind the line ("in the kitchen"), the 7-ball is on the foot spot, and the 8-ball is on the rail a diamond from the corner pocket. You can shoot a finesse shot with slow speed and try to die at A for position, or you can use an aggressive stroke with low right English and leave the cueball near C. Top players are deadly on this, the so-called spot shot, and most of them would fire the 7-ball in with draw as diagrammed. The soft shot, while feasible, requires delicate speed control to get an easy shot on the black.

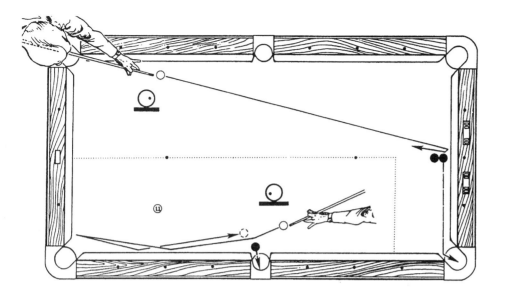

95 Rail first to score and double-the-rail for position

Consider the shot in the upper portion of the diagram. Cutting the far black ball into the corner from such a distance and at such an angle is difficult, but making it rail first is easy. The shot comes up frequently in line-up straight pool when you've run the table but left the cueball at the wrong end of the table. (See Section 16, Rules of Major Pool Games, at the end of Book One.)

At the bottom is a position maneuver that never seems to occur to some players. Say the game is 14.1 straight pool, the balls are to be racked at the left end of the table, and the shooter wants to cut the black in the side and get rack-breaking position on the 11. The elegant method in the diagram is called doubling the rail. It's a simple maneuver that always evokes a pleased reaction from the spectators.

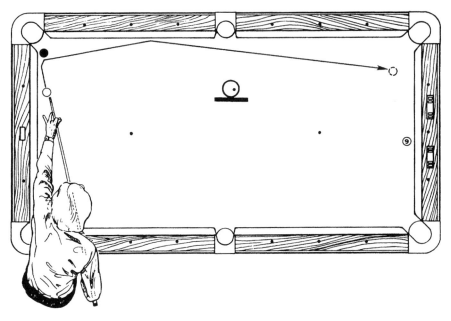

96 Rail first for position with English

How can the black ball be pocketed and good position be obtained on the 9 at the other end of the table? By using right English and hitting the rail first. The shot is so easy and comes up so often that you must learn to execute it with deadly precision. Beginners will soon learn that if the cueball is a foot or two to the right to start with, much less speed is needed for the same result.

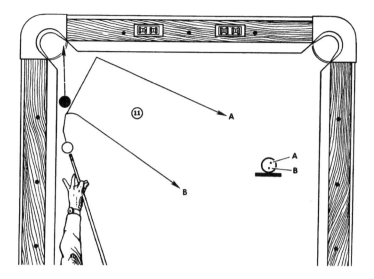

97 Rail first for position with follow and draw

The black ball is straight in. The player wants to make it and get the cueball to an area from which the 11 can be sent into the same pocket. (Interfering balls that rule out other goals are omitted for simplicity.) Two courses are open. Rail first with draw brings the cueball to B. Rail first with follow and right English sends it to A. Follow without right is risky because the cueball might come off the end rail too steeply and come to rest on the wrong side of the 11.

Rail-first shots are easy when the object ball is within a half-inch of the rail; think twice when the gap is wider.

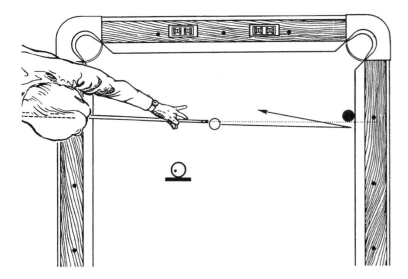

98 The "impossible" cut shot

The dotted line is drawn from the edge of the black ball at right angles to the rail. Since the cueball overlaps the line, it would seem that the required contact point on the black ball is inaccessible—it is, on a direct line. The trick is to hit the rail first with plenty of left English. If the cueball barely misses the black on the way in, it will clip it just right on the way out (the action is too fast to see), and the black will glide mysteriously into the pocket. A hard stroke must be used, and the cueball can be all the way across the line. Set it up as a challenge. Win money.

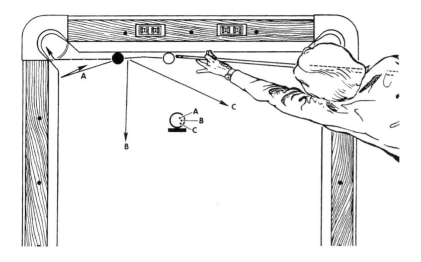

99 Sinking into the rail for position

To serious players who don't already know it, and their numbers are legion, this shot is worth the price of the book. The object ball and cueball are frozen to the rail, yet the ball can be made and the cueball sent to any part of the table. To do it, hit the cueball on the right side and aim slightly into the rail instead of directly at the black. The cueball compresses the rubber and hits the black at a slight angle. Right English must be used to make sure that the cue tip doesn't interfere with the cueball as it emerges from the rubber. Again, the action is too fast to see.

Things to remember: 1. The farther the two balls are apart, the harder the cueball must be hit and the less pronounced should be the into-the-rail angle; 2. Don't shoot into the rail if the balls are more than a diamond apart; 3. The closer the balls are together the easier the shot is and the more positional freedom the player has; 4. It is not nice to win money if the loser can't afford it.

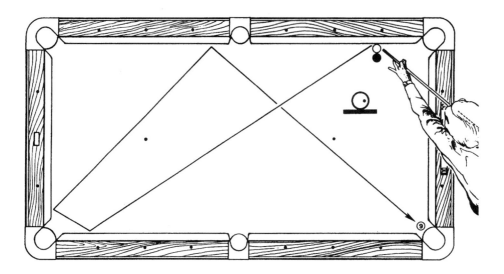

100 Sinking into the rail to avoid interference

I've never been in this pickle, but if I ever am, I'll be ready. The 9 is in the jaws and the black has the cueball pinned against the rail. Thrill your loved ones by shooting hard into the rail at slightly less than a 45-degree angle with right English. The cueball will sink into the rubber and escape without touching the black. With practice you can make the cueball travel around the table as shown and pocket the 9-ball more often than not. Try it first without the interfering ball.

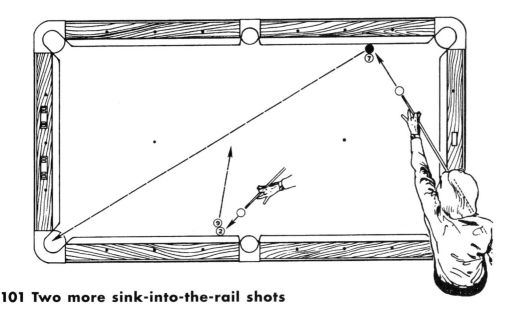

101 Two more sink-into-the-rail shots

At the upper right is a shot closely related to the previous one. The challenge is to bank the black ball into the corner without touching or moving the 7. It only looks impossible.

At the bottom of the diagram, the 2 is frozen to the rail a half-diamond from the side pocket and the 9 is frozen to the 2. The line of centers is aimed at the second diamond on the opposite rail. By hitting the 2 flush in the face, the 9 will go across the table at an unexpected angle, possibly into the side pocket. The angle of the 9's path depends on how deeply the 2 is forced into the cushion.

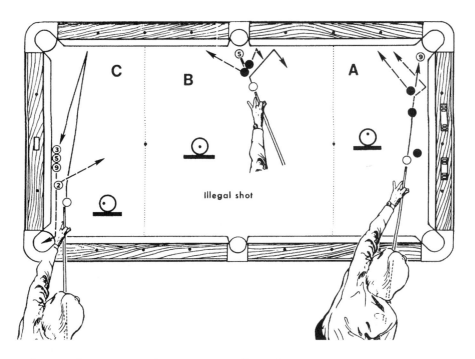

Illegal shot

102 Three clearance shots—one illegal

Making a clearance shot in a game is a profound pleasure that comes to few human beings. In A, your path to the 9-ball seems hopelessly blocked, while behind your back your smirking opponent awaits the kill. Then! You see an exquisite shot lying there waiting to be made! You shoot straight ahead with follow, the two black balls carom out of the way, the cueball continues forward in a straight line to pocket the 9, and your opponent skewers himself on his cue.

B can be made in similar fashion. There is an easier, illegal way, however, that is not recommended unless everyone has been smoking unorthodox cigarettes. Plant your left hand close to the cueball and shoot straight at the 5. The black balls will split, the cueball will careen to the right, and by using a long follow-through, you can knock the 5 in with your cue tip.

C is another one of those shots that can be used to win a bet in a bar. The challenge is to make the 9-ball, which seems hopelessly trapped by other balls. The secret is to bank the 2 out of the way and, with the aid of left English, bring the cueball off the rail into the 3.

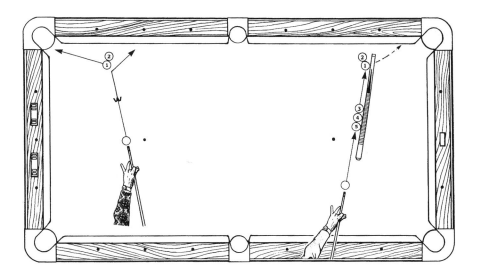

103 A carom subtlety

At the left, the 1-ball is frozen to the 2 in a way that makes pocketing the 1 in the corner a cinch. All you have to do is hit the right side of the 1 at any speed and in it goes. But let's say the 1 is at point W instead of frozen to the 2. If you drive the 1 into the 2 so it hits the same contact point on the 2, the 1 won't go unless you shoot hard. Why? Because in traveling a foot or two across the cloth, the 1 picks up forward roll, and after the carom the topspin will make the path of the 1 curve into the rail.

Proof is at the right. Begin by using the butt of a cue to position the 1, 3, 4, and 5 in a straight line. Next, freeze the 2 against the 1 so that the carom line is the same as the shot at the left, in other words, make it a dead carom shot. Finally, remove the 1-ball. If you drive the cueball into the 5 as diagrammed, the 3 will hit the 2 at the precise point at which the 1 was frozen to the 2. But at medium speeds the 3 won't carom off the 2 into the corner; instead it will curve forward and hit the rail (dashed line). It will seem as if the 3 hit the 2 too thinly, but that's an optical illusion. Only if you use enough speed to cause the 3 to *slide* into the 2 will the 3 travel in a straight line to the pocket.

The lesson to be learned is simple. Unless the object balls on a carom shot are touching or nearly touching, use plenty of speed.

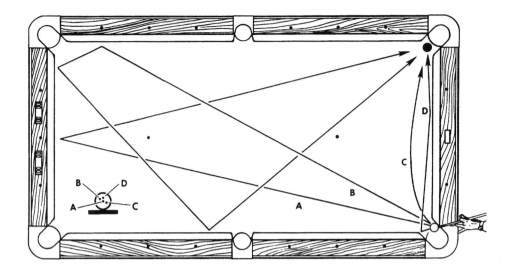

104 Four ways to escape a "corner hook"

When the cueball comes to rest on the lip of a corner pocket, putting the point of the cushion between you and the object ball, all is not necessarily lost. Place the balls as diagrammed and there are four ways to make the black ball. A is a one-rail bank with a centerball hit, B is a three-cushion bank with running English, C is a difficult massé with right English and a steeply elevated cue, and D is a bank off the opposite side of the corner pocket. Many supposedly well-educated people are ignorant of D.

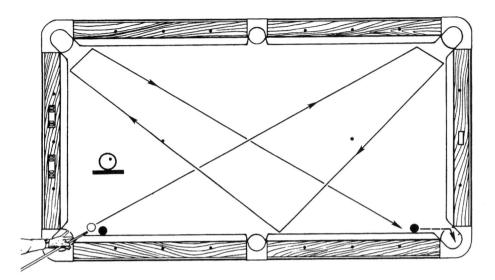

105 Five rails first to escape interference

Willie Mosconi said he once won a world championship with this shot. Trapped behind one ball, he made the other with a five-rail-first bank. Pulling this off in a game would be truly amazing, but it's not so tough when you can put the balls where you want them and practice it a few times.

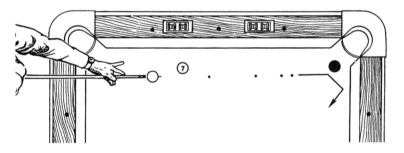

106 The jump shot

The black ball is hidden behind the edge of the 7. A massé could be tried, but a jump shot is far more secure. Elevate the cue to an angle of 20 or 30 degrees and strike the cueball a hair above center. (It is a foul to golf the ball into the air by hitting underneath it.) In the diagram the dots are intended to show where the cueball touches the table as it bounces toward the corner.

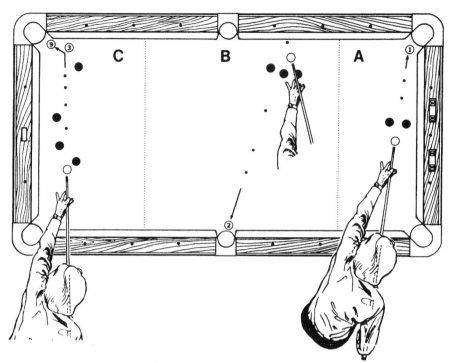

107 Three more jump shots

At the right is a shot beloved by exhibition players because it seems to require great skill. It is, in fact, laughably easy. Freeze the cueball between two object balls, then move it six inches away. Is it possible to shoot through a space precisely the width of a ball without touching either black ball and make the one in the corner? Yes, by shooting into the cueball at a slightly downward angle. The cueball is in the air as it passes through the gap, which can't be detected.

Shot B is spectacular and dangerous. Elevate the cue, shoot crisply downward, and the cueball in rebounding from the cushion will vault the picket fence and cross the table to pocket the 2-ball . . . it will, that is, if you know what you are doing. If you don't, you will break a window and injure the moppets outside.

In shot C it would be asking too much even of Evel Knievel to jump over two balls to make the 9. A carom off the 3, though, after a modest hop over the edge of one interfering ball, is easy.

Reference: See When and How to Shoot Jump Shots in *Byrne's Advanced Technique.*

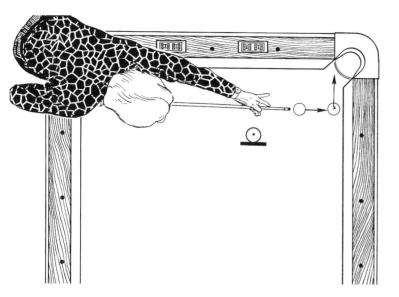

108 The coin-op smother shot

If the cueball is larger and heavier than the object ball, as it is on most coin-op tavern tables, the game is altered in many ways. It's harder to draw the cueball, though easier to follow. Making an object ball that's frozen to a rail is slightly harder if the cueball is bigger. Perfect stop shots are harder. Carom angles aren't quite what you expect if you are used to playing with balls of equal weight.

On the other hand, there are several shots that are possible only if the cueball is heavier than the object ball, such as the one diagrammed above. Because a heavy cueball immediately moves forward when hitting a light object ball, the ball on the rail can be "smothered" or double-kissed into the corner pocket. The shot is impossible with balls of equal weight.

Reference: For more, including an explanation of an ingenious combination shot, see Coping with the Heavy Tavern Cueball in *Byrne's Advanced Technique.*

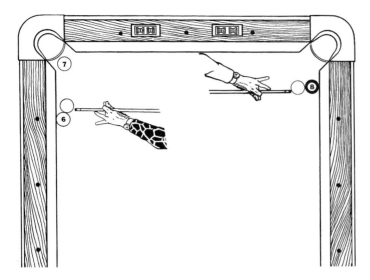

109 Two dubious rail shots

These two frozen rail shots are intended for amusement purposes only. Don't try them in a game unless your opponent is considerably smaller than you are, is momentarily distracted, or doesn't know right from wrong. At the right, as unlikely as it may seem, the 8-ball can be made in the corner pocket, though not without suspicion. Position the cue tip against the cueball right of center as shown and push, don't stroke. Meshed like cogwheels, both balls will move to the left.

Bill Marshall learned the devilish shot at the left from the late, great Luther "Wimpy" Lassiter. I call it Wimpy's Pinch. With extreme left English, move the cue forward in a slow, controlled manner so that the tip hits the cueball again, miscuing it to the right to pocket the 7-ball. You'll need half a dozen tries to get the hang of it.

Reference: More frozen rail shots can be found in the section called Twenty-five Easy Ones in *Byrne's Treasury of Trick Shots* and in *Byrne's Standard Video of Trick Shots, Vol. III.* See the video for a demonstration of Wimpy's Pinch.

9

analyzing clusters

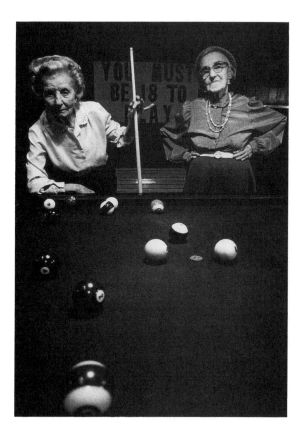

(Photo copyright by Tim Bieber)

Recognizing shots when they are presented in isolation is one thing and picking them out of a crowd is another. If you have trouble doing it, then we've found another facet of your game that needs polishing. The diagrams in this section will give you practice in uncovering shots that are hidden in random arrays. Do your best before reading the answers in the accompanying text.

(The arrays aren't random, of course . . . they are contrived for teaching purposes. In real life there may be no shot.)

To make the nine positions intellectually challenging, I've used large clusters of the type that occur most often in games like 14.1 straight pool and one-pocket, which don't begin with open breaks. In each case, there is a ball that can be pocketed fairly easily. You can hit any ball first.

Pull off shots like these in games and applause will ring in your ears.

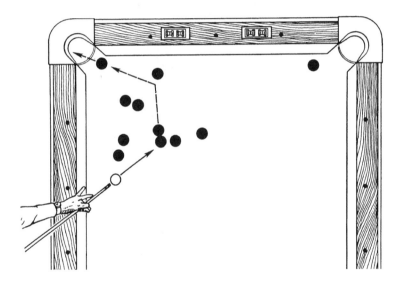

110 An apparently hopeless bunch of balls

If you were confronted with this mess, would you see the combination-carom shot? Note that the first black ball must be hit squarely to throw the second one to the right; otherwise the carom on the third ball will be too thin.

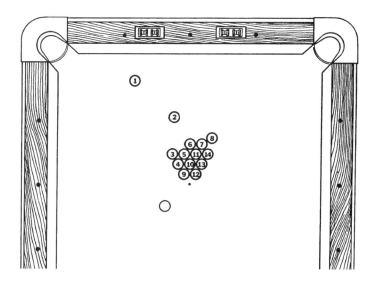

111 What's the best shot? Position 1

Don't read this until you've made a guess. The first thing an experienced player would notice is that the 8 can be thrown into the corner if the 7 can be hit on the proper side. The 11, therefore, is the right "third ball" (see Diagram 65), not the 6. Everything depends on whether or not the 9, 10, 11, and 7 are frozen together. If they are, all you need to do is hit the 9 head on—the force will be transmitted instantaneously to the 7 through the 11. You must lean over the table and study the cluster closely. If there are small gaps in the chain, the shot is uncertain because the force might be transmitted to the 7 by way of the 4, 5, and 6, which would throw the 8 to the right, away from the pocket. There is another problem if the 9, 10, 11, and 7 aren't frozen tightly together—force will be spent in moving other balls. If the 9 has to be hit hard to get enough power through to the 7, a ball like the 14 might bank off the side rail and get in the way.

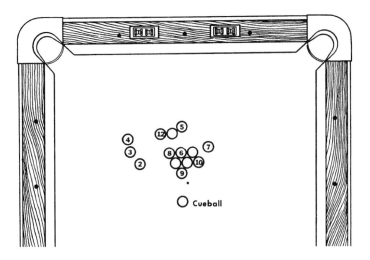

112 What's the best shot? Position 2

Carom the cueball off the 2 into the 12 and the 5 will go. Many shots like this are easy once you see them.

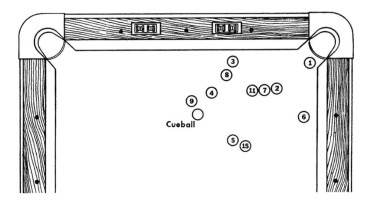

113 What's the best shot? Position 3

You might overlook this one among the red herrings. Shoot into the left side of the 6, drawing the cueball into the 1.

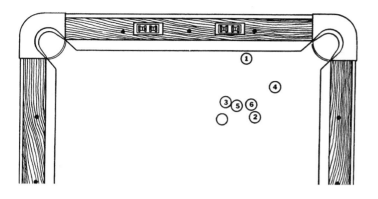

114 What's the best shot? Position 4

Give up? Hit the 2 head on, banking it into the 6. From that direction the 3 is dead. Don't let the cueball follow forward and interfere with the 2 as it comes off the rail.

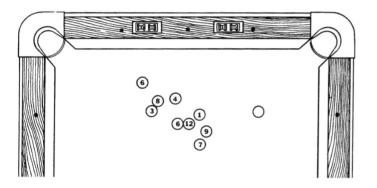

115 What's the best shot? Position 5

The 3 will kiss off the 8 into the corner pocket if you can get it started. Knocking the 1-ball into the 12 is no good because the 6 will be thrown to the left and will miss the 3 entirely. Cut the 9 into the 12 and all is well.

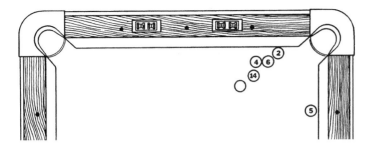

116 What's the best shot? Position 6

None of these positions may ever come up in your own games, at least not precisely, but that is not the point. The point is to alert you to certain pregnancies. Here the 4-6 pair is parallel to the rail, which means that the 4 can be thrown into the left corner pocket if the 6 can be hit on the proper side. The cueball can't be banked directly into the 6 because the 14 is in the way, so bring it back off the left side of the 5. Use low left English.

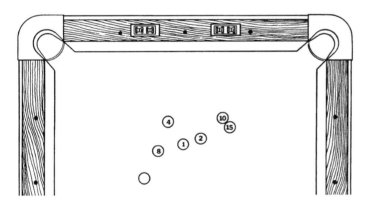

117 What's the best shot? Position 7

It might be possible to carom the 8 off the 4 into the corner, but it would be delicate. Why try that when there is something easier? Carom the 8 off the 4 into the 10.

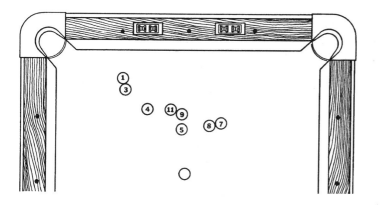

118 What's the best shot? Position 8

This one is hard to see. If you could approach the 1-ball from the direction of the left corner pocket it would be easy to send it into the right corner pocket because it is resting against the 3 at exactly the right angle. Easiest is the two-cushion-first bank. Aim the cueball a few inches to the left of the left pocket with right English.

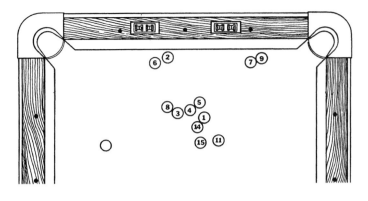

119 What's the best shot? Position 9

On the other hand, don't be reckless, either. Almost all of the drawings in this book are of shots that can be made, but real life is not so accommodating. Quite often there is no shot on the table worth trying, and defensive play must be resorted to. Cluster shots are especially dangerous because they often break the game open for one player or the other. Don't spread the balls unless you are quite sure of the shot.

In the diagram, the 9 will go if the 7 can be struck on the side closest the rail. Carom the cueball off the right side of the 6 or the 2. The target presented by the left side of the 7 is rather large because the cueball can hit the rail just before the 7.

Reference: If you like challenges of this sort, see the book *How Would You Play This?* by George Fels (Contemporary Books, Chicago, 1998).

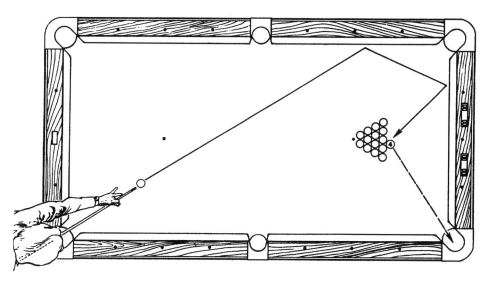

120 A cluster trick shot

Set this one up and see if anybody can figure out a way to make the 4. The secret is a two-rail-first bank. You'll need a few trial runs to find the spot to shoot for on the first rail. Use right English.

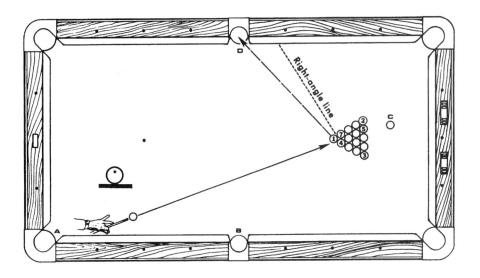

121 The ultimate cluster shot

Is there a shot that can be called from the full rack? Not with any confidence. In games requiring the ball and pocket to be called, it is crazy to try to score on the opening break unless you are playing just for fun or against a patsy.

If you insist on spreading the balls for your opponent by taking goofy chances, the best bet from behind the line is probably the 1-ball in the side. If you can induce backspin on the 1 by putting follow on the cueball, the 1 will diverge from the right-angle line as shown and will drop into the side pocket every once in a while.

Another low-percentage but not impossible shot from the same starting point is the length-of-the-table 3-ball bank into corner pocket A. Use a half-ball hit and left English.

The 2 can sometimes be banked in the side from cueball position C.

One of "Machine Gun" Lou Butera's exhibition shots is the 4-ball in side pocket B from cueball position C. Shoot between the 2 and the 5, but don't hit them simultaneously. If the 2 is touched first, the 1 will move slightly before the 4 kisses off it.

People who try over and over again to make the corner balls go directly into the corner pockets, from whatever cueball position, should consider switching to hobbies that don't require so much self-control. Bowling is a nice game.

10

how to run the table

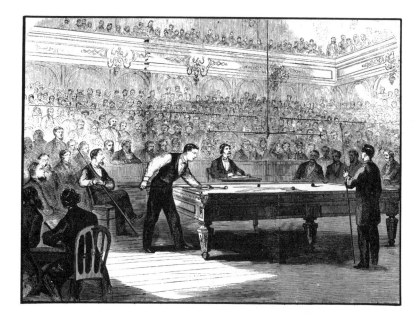

The first tournament held in the United States.
(*Harper's Weekly*, 1863; The Billiard Archive)

Running the table in any pool game takes skill, practice, concentration, foresight, a grasp of what we've covered so far, and more. The "more" includes gaining an angle, visualizing the position zone, leaving an insurance shot, moving trouble balls, separating clusters, and picking the right sequence of shots, all of which we'll take up now.

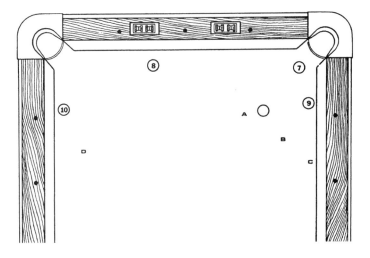

122 Gaining an angle—the key to high runs

To run more than two balls it's not enough to make the first and get position on the second—you must get a *certain kind* of position. In the diagram, what's the best way to make the 7, 8, 9, and 10 in numerical order? A stop shot on the 7 is fine if the 8-ball is the limit of your greed, but if you want *all* the balls you must "gain an angle" on the 8. Otherwise it's too tough to get from the 8 to the 9. Shoot the 7 with draw, pulling the cueball back to point A. Now with low right English the 8 can be made and the cueball brought to B or thereabouts. C is bad because there is no angle on the 9. From B it's a simple matter to pocket the 9 and send the cueball to D for the 10.

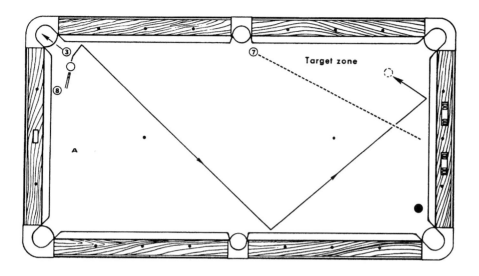

Target zone

123 Gaining an angle—another example

In a game of eight-ball you find yourself with the 3 and the 7 left. The black ball is your opponent's. How can you make your two balls and get position on the 8 to win the game? The easiest way is to make the 3 and gain an angle on the 7. All you have to do is make sure the cueball reaches the triangular area marked by the dashed line, from which it will be no problem to cut the 7 in the side and leave the cueball near the left end rail for the 8.

Anybody who can't reach a target zone as big as the one required here should be ashamed of himself. If you are afraid of scratching in the side, you can draw the cueball off the 3 along the upper long rail; the danger is touching the 7 as you pass it, which might spoil everything.

The black ball prevents trying for the position pattern shown in Diagram 81.

The concept of gaining an angle is sometimes called three-ball planning. If you have three or more balls to make, you must think three shots ahead. First is the shot at hand, second is the ball you are playing position on, and third is the next one. You won't make the third ball unless you get the right kind of angle on the second one.

Good practice is to throw three balls onto the table, then place the cueball by hand in a place that enables you to make them in numerical order. When that becomes too easy, throw out four or five or six. Figuring out where to place the cueball to start is excellent exercise for the brain.

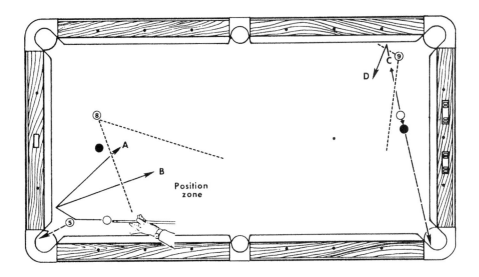

124 How to enter the position zone

Because a target is easier to hit when you know where it is, it's often helpful to imagine the limits of the desired position zone. At the left, the shooter needs only to cut the 5 in and get position on the 8 to win the game. Anywhere between the dashed lines is OK. Once the shooter realizes that the position zone is triangular, he will see the danger of trying for point A—crossing the narrow neck of the triangle requires too much precision in speed control. Hitting less 5-ball or using a touch of hold-up English (left in this case) directs the cueball along a line that has a much greater margin of error.

At the right is a position from a game of nine-ball. The goal is to pocket the black ball and draw back for position on the 9. C requires too much precision. Better to use a lot of draw, rebounding smartly off the rail into the broad part of the position zone.

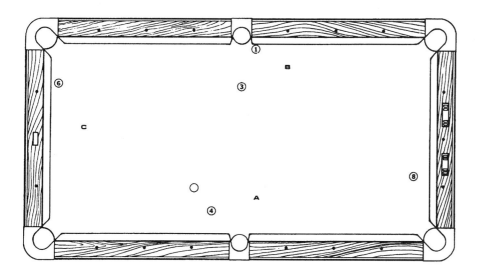

125 Moving the "trouble" ball

Now and then you will have a table that can rather easily be cleared, except for one inconveniently located ball. In the diagram, such a ball is the 1. Fortunately, it can be bumped to a better place. If the 1, 3, and 8 are the only ones left in a game of eight-ball, shoot a stop shot on the 3, caroming it into the side off the 1, and knocking the 1 a couple of feet to the right. If the 4 and 6 are also on the table, there are several possible strategies. One is to make the 4, using high left to get to point A, thus gaining an angle on the 3. Pocket the 3 off the 1, sending the cueball to C. Depending on where the 1 came to rest, make the 6 with whatever speed and English are necessary.

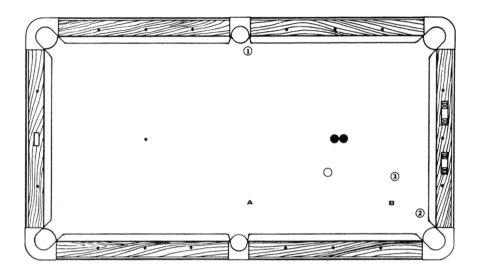

126 Breaking up "trouble" clusters

Common is an array of balls with one "trouble" cluster. The player must devote his attention toward gaining the right kind of angle on one of the loose balls. A solution to the problem posed in the diagram is to cut the 2 and leave the cueball at A; from there the 1 can be cut in the side and the cueball sent into the cluster. Some players might try a soft stroke on the 2, hoping for a break off the 3 from point B. Two drawbacks with that approach are that B has a smaller margin of error than A, and that from B the cluster will be broken toward an obstructed pocket. Because it is hard to predict how clusters will spread, it is usually wise to delay breaks until interfering balls are removed.

Small clusters like this one need only be nudged. Save your power for big packs.

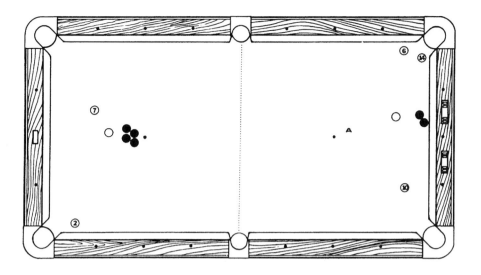

127 Leaving an insurance shot

At the left side of the diagram, two balls are loose and four are stuck together. Shooting a stop shot on the 7 and breaking the cluster off the 2 is taking an unnecessary step into the unknown. It is better to draw the cueball from the 7 into the cluster. Draw is a poor way to approach a large group of balls, but three or four can usually be spread sufficiently. The point here is that no matter what happens after the draw from the 7, the 2 is waiting as insurance against disaster.

    At the right, it is possible to make the 14 and draw the cueball into the cluster, but there is a safer course. Make the 10 and leave the cueball at A. Cut the 6 and use right English to direct the cueball into the black balls. If the cueball gets locked up, the 14 will bail you out.

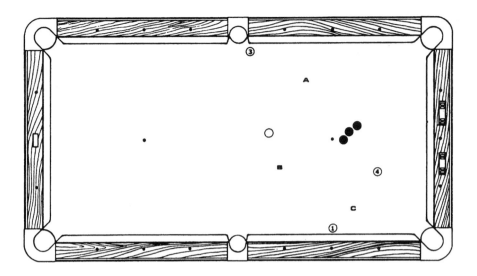

128 When to leave clusters alone

Some clusters are benign rather than malignant. They may contain makable combinations or kiss shots and it may be possible to chip away at them ball by ball. In the diagram, the black balls are trouble only as long as the side and corner pockets are blocked by the 3 and 4. A hyperactive child might try to break the black balls apart at once by cutting the 1 in the corner, trusting to luck for the next shot. There are saner courses. One is to cut the 3 into the side and leave the cueball at C for the 4 or for one of the black balls in the side. Another is to start by cutting the 4 into the corner, leaving the cueball at A. Another is to run the 1 down the rail and leave the cueball near the cluster for the 4.

Running the table—thirteen rules to live by

1. Because a ball frozen on a rail can usually be approached from only one side and made easily in only one pocket, look for chances to make such shots early in the run.

2. If you have a choice among several balls, take the one that clears the way for other balls.

3. Beware of breaking a cluster toward an obstructed pocket.

4. If it's not too much trouble, wait until most loose balls around a cluster are gone before you break it; otherwise you might create a new cluster.

5. Think twice before breaking a cluster on a low-percentage shot because if you miss and spread the cluster you have solved your opponent's problem instead of your own. Think safety instead.

6. Break small clusters lightly.

7. Look for opportunities to break clusters when there is an insurance shot.

8. Try not to bump into balls that are already separated to avoid forming new clusters.

9. Don't risk missing in order to get perfect position on the next ball. Better to cinch the shot and get so-so position, which still leaves you with the option of playing safe.

10. Try to send the cueball into a cluster at a point that will most likely spread the balls advantageously.

11. When you can easily do so, avoid the narrow end of the position zone.

12. Think three shots ahead.

13. Have a plan, but reevaluate it after every shot.

the keys to winning eight-ball

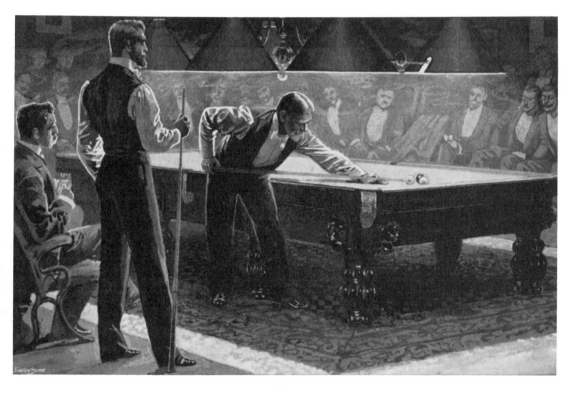

A serious game: Nursing the balls.
From *Billiards*, by Major W. Broadfoot, R.E.
Longmans, Green and Co., London and Bombay, 1896
Illustrated by Lucien Davies, R.I.

America's favorite cue game

Far more pool is played in taverns and homes—where the game of choice is eight-ball—than in public rooms or private clubs. Eight-ball is easily the most popular pool game, and many casual players are familiar with no other. Disdained by professionals as too short and simple to be a proper test of skill, the game nevertheless contains a wealth of strategic subtleties.

The best feature of eight-ball is that it lends itself to come-from-behind rallies. If a player misses after running five or six balls, the other player often has the advantage because he has more options and more ways to play safe. The lesson is plain: Never leave an impossible cluster or a low-percentage shot till the end, for then you will likely miss and leave a wide-open table for your hated opponent.

The worst feature of the game is that the rules differ from one league to another, from one tavern to another, sometimes even from one player to another in the same tavern. Make sure you know the rules before making an unfriendly wager. Do you win or lose if you make the 8-ball on the break? After a foul or a scratch, can the cueball be placed anywhere on the table or must it be placed behind the line? Is it OK to play safe without trying to make a ball? Do illegally pocketed balls stay down or are they respotted? What 8-ball fouls lose the game? Arguments over such questions can turn ugly, it is my sad duty to report.

The keys to winning eight-ball relate to choosing the right group, handling problem clusters, playing safe, and recognizing key balls. Because the possibilities are infinite, it's easy to dream up examples by the dozens, by the hundreds, by the thousands. The diagrams that follow are designed to show you the kind of thought processes that are required. When two players of equal technical ability face each other, the superior problem solver will be the winner.

My sympathy if you must play under rules that don't allow deliberate safeties, for a whole world of cleverness and skill is lost. Campaign for peaceful change.

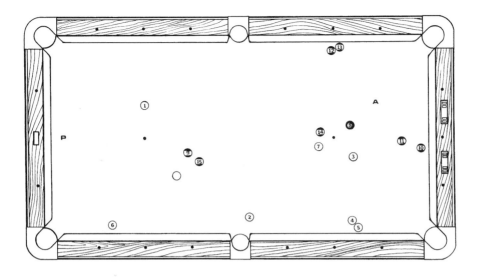

129 Choosing the right group

Your opponent broke and nothing dropped. It's up to you to make a ball and establish the groups for the rest of the game. If only one group has a problem cluster, the choice is easy, but here each group has a cluster that must be broken. The cueball is close to the 9-ball, so a possibility is to pocket the 9 in the side with follow and send the cueball off one rail to the vicinity of A, from which point you might be able to make the 11 or 10 and draw back to split the 12-13 cluster.

Better is to choose the solids instead of the stripes. Make the 1-ball and leave the cueball near the middle of the table. From there it's easy to make the 2-ball and send the cueball lightly into the 4 and 5. Soft speed is best to avoid forming new clusters with the nearby balls. You'll almost certainly be left with a good shot on the 4, 5, 3, or 7.

But let's say that after separating the 4 and 5 you have nothing but a long, straight shot at the 6-ball. Let's say further that the only way to continue the run is to pocket the 6 and draw back three or four feet—pretty hard from long range, especially if the cueball is heavier than the 6. An option to consider in such a case is a deliberate miss. Hit the 6 thin and leave the cueball on the rail at P. Even if your opponent gets lucky and makes the long, tough 14-ball in the upper right corner, he still has the 12-13 problem to worry about while all the balls in your group are in the clear.

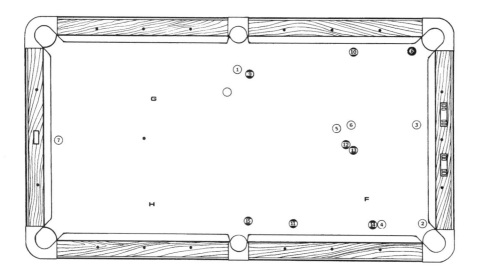

130 Another choice of groups

All the balls are on the table and it's your shot. Stripes or solids? The 14-ball and the 11 pose a problem, as does the 10, which is blocked by the 8. I'd pick the spots despite the 4-14 cluster and the 7 at the far end. Here's one way to proceed: Pocket the 1 in the side and bump 9 toward the 10 and the blocked pocket. Cut the 2 in and with slight right sidespin send the cueball lightly into the 4, freeing it and knocking the 14 toward the 11, possibly creating another problem for your opponent. But what if the cueball drifts too far after making the 1, leaving you with no direct shot at the 2? Consider banking the 3 toward the middle of the table while caroming the cueball off the 3 into the 2. Instead you could hit the 4 thinly and softly, freeing it from the 14 and leaving the cueball against the 2. You have yielded the table, but if your opponent can't "see" the 15, you are in a very strong position.

Assume you have made the 1 and the 2, broken the 4 loose, and left the cueball near the letter F. What then? If the 3 will go by the 8, take it and try for position on the 6 in the side. If the 3 won't go, and if there is no shot on the 4, there are two safety plays to consider. One is to bump the 3 or the 4 to better positions while leaving no shot. The other is to shoot the length of the table to the left side of the 7-ball, banking it to the vicinity of G while leaving the cueball near H.

Aggressive safeties of this type, which solve a problem or improve your overall chances of running out later, are powerful offensive weapons. Recognizing them can determine the best group to select.

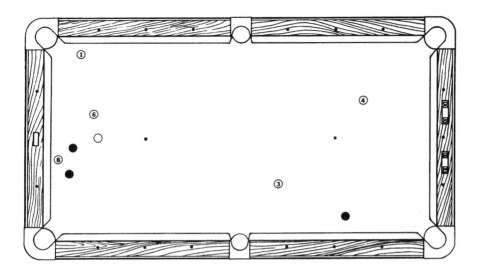

131 The principle of the key ball

If a critical play must be made, the ball that makes it possible is called the key ball. In the diagrammed position, the shooter must make the 1, 3, 4, and 6 followed by the 8-ball. The black balls are from the other group. Note that the 8 is hemmed in and can only be approached along a narrow avenue. It would be a monstrous blunder to make the 6 first and then the 1 because the 1 is the key to position on the 8. Correct is to make the 6 using high right English to send the cueball one rail to the center of the table or a little beyond. After pocketing the 3 and the 4, it is a simple matter to make the 1 and then the 8.

In Diagram 129, the 2-ball is the key to breaking the 4-5 cluster, so it should not be pocketed until it can be used for that purpose. Sometimes it is worth spending a shot to create a key ball by knocking it to a good place.

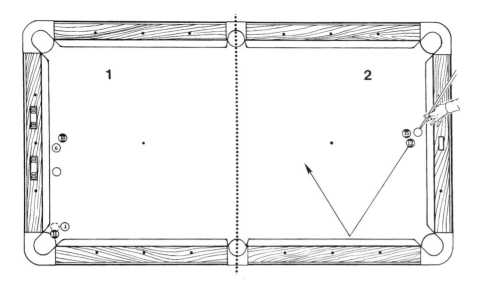

132 Devilish safety plays—I

On rare occasions, it is advantageous to pocket one of your opponent's balls. In shot 1, left, you have the solids. The corner pocket is blocked by a stripe and you have a problem cluster, the 6-10, to contend with as well. (Other balls have been omitted for clarity.) There is a way to seize the initiative in sensational fashion. Hit the 6 squarely, sending it and the 10 down the table, and draw the cueball back to make the 11-ball. You can step away from the table confidently, for your opponent is locked up tight against the 3-ball and helpless. In some positions of this type—without a problem cluster to break up, for example—a similar safety can be achieved by simply pocketing the 11 softly after grazing the 3.

In shot 2, right, you have ball in hand after a foul and can place the ball anywhere on the table. You are shooting the stripes and the rest of the balls are at the other end of the table. A good place to put the cueball is behind the two-ball problem cluster as shown. Bank the 12-ball toward the center of the table and leave the cueball snug against the 15. You have eliminated the cluster and left your opponent in jail without a prayer. Warning! You will be in jail yourself if you accidentally bank the 12 in the side. I've witnessed many such tragedies.

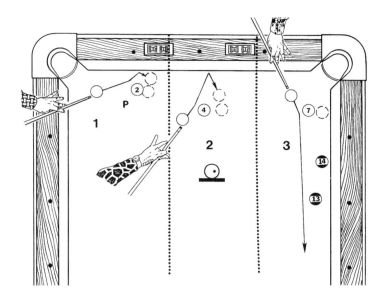

133 Devilish safety plays—II

Shot 1: You have left yourself straight in on the 2-ball and can't get to the other end of the table . . . or maybe you have ball in hand and want to play a safety. A thin hit on the 2 with very soft speed will leave the balls in the position of the dashed circles. Be sure to hit the ball first, because a legal shot requires the cueball or an object ball to hit a rail after the initial collision. If you also have one of your balls at point P, another stratagem comes into view. Announce that you are playing safe and pocket the 2-ball with a stop shot. The 2 stays down and your opponent must shoot from a terrible position.

Shot 2: Same as shot 1 but tougher. You'll need practice to find out how to blend speed, sidespin, and thinness of hit to leave the cueball behind the object ball.

Shot 3: It's a big advantage if one or more of your opponent's balls are blocked by the 8-ball or one of your balls because a run-out is difficult. If you feel your opponent can't run out, you have the luxury of spending your turn at the table breaking one of your problem clusters open or knocking one of your balls to the mouth of a pocket. In the diagram, a thin hit on the 7-ball will leave it on the rail and block two balls. You can make the 7 later when the time is right.

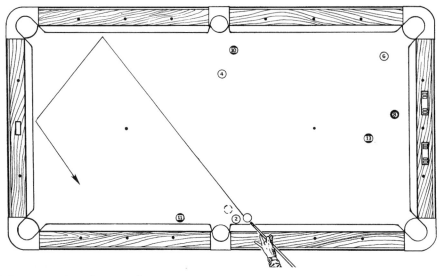

134 An aggressive safety

A passive safety is a legal shot that denies your opponent an opening and leaves you no worse than you were. Much to be preferred is an aggressive safety, a shot that improves your position or makes your opponent's worse. Diagrammed is a simple example of an aggressive safety. In trying to run out the game, you accidentally bumped the 2-ball against the rail. What now? The 4 and the 6 are easy shots but do nothing to solve the problem of the 2-ball. A strong move is to hit the 2 extremely thin, nudging it in front of the side pocket (dashed circle) and driving the cueball two rails. Leaving the cueball in the vicinity of the arrowhead forces your sweating adversary to try the difficult cut of the 13 into the upper right corner with no control of the cueball.

Does it go against your grain to be defensive when you have open shots? Then you could ignore my advice and try to be a hero (and probably fail) by starting with a stop shot on the 4-ball. Next, cut the 6 in and try to send the cueball one rail into the 2. If you fail to hit the 2—or if you hit it and are left without a reasonable shot on it—*then* play a safety. Trouble is, with the 4 and 6 off the table, your opponent can easily return the safety and possibly leave you with nothing.

How to win at eight-ball—a checklist

1. If you have a choice of groups and both have problem clusters, pick the group that has a ball that can be pocketed (a "key" ball) while the cueball spreads the cluster.
2. Other things being equal, choose the group that will enable you to spread a cluster with a safety shot.
3. Don't try to run out unless you are pretty sure you can. Running down to the last ball or two and then missing is usually a disaster.
4. Try not to pocket a key ball before its time.
5. Improve your position, if you can do so with safety, by using your turn to move a problem ball, create a key ball, spread a problem cluster, or bury the cueball behind one of your balls.
6. Think twice before making a ball that interferes with balls from the other group.
7. Try low-percentage shots only when you think your opponent can't run out if you miss.
8. Consider missing on purpose if leaving one of your balls in front of a pocket blocks one or more of your opponent's balls.
9. If you have only one good shot and the angle is wrong for position, knock the ball to a better place if you can do it without selling out.
10. Watch for chances to make a ball and at the same time create a problem for your opponent—by bumping, for example, one of his balls against one that is on a rail.
11. If all your balls are in the clear and you decide to try for a run-out, don't let the cueball hit other balls and risk forming a problem cluster.
12. Above all, make sure safety play is allowed under local rules!

the keys to winning nine-ball

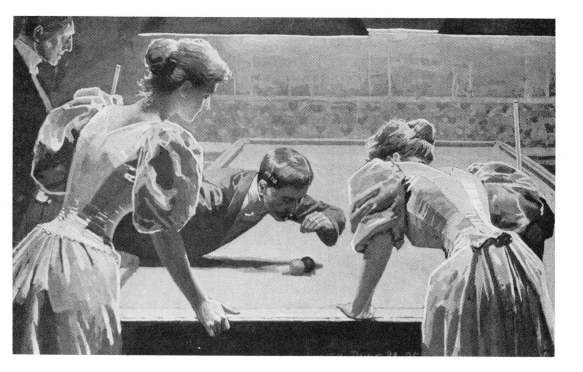

Are they touching?
From *Billiards,* by Major W. Broadfoot, R.E.
Longmans, Green and Co., London and Bombay, 1896
Illustrated by Lucien Davies, R.I.

The nine-ball juggernaut

Over the last thirty-five years or so, it's remarkable how nine-ball has taken over as the premier tournament game for pro and semipro players. Once thought of mainly as a gambling game, it's now virtually the only cue game ever shown on television. Before the 1960s, 14.1 straight pool was the game of choice for major tournaments. But straight pool, in which it is seldom necessary to move the cueball more than a few feet—a few inches often suffices—and which sometimes bogs down in long safety exchanges, is not the best spectator game, nor is it well suited to the small screen. Good position players seem never to face a tough shot and their long runs can appear mechanical and uninspiring.

Nine-ball is a far better television game. Players are forced to try tough shots and move the cueball all over the table. It has become so popular—partly because of television—that it is now often played on coin-op tavern tables where eight-ball once ruled unchallenged.

The rules are deceptively simple. The balls are numbered 1 through 9. The cueball must always hit the lowest-numbered ball first, though the balls need not be pocketed in numerical order. If you hit the low ball and any ball goes in, you shoot again. Whoever makes the 9-ball on a legal shot, at any point in the game, wins.

To be a consistent winner at nine-ball, you need to be good at bank shots, long shots, jump shots, and curve shots. You need to be a good long-roll position player, a good safety player, and a good escape artist. By the latter I mean you must be able to bank the cueball off one or more rails to hit the lowest ball. Because the penalty for all fouls is ball-in-hand anywhere on the table, and because three fouls in a row means loss of game, skill at playing safe and getting out of safeties is essential.

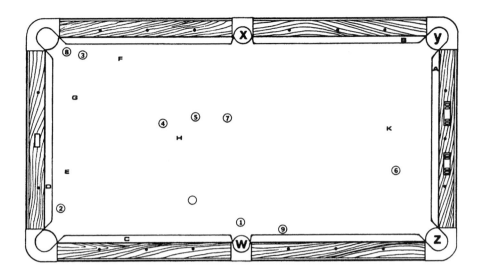

135 A nine-ball run-out

Running the table in nine-ball is a laudable feat because the balls must be taken in numerical order. In the above position, many lower-echelon players would slam the 1 into the 9, hoping that by "giving the 9 a ride" it will drop in pocket Z, or somewhere. Professionals, noting that the balls are well spread, would try to run out instead. The first problem is making the 1 and getting position on the 2. Cut the 1 thinly enough to make it and use low left English to send the cueball off the rails at points A, B, C, D, and E. E is not ideal because there is no way to reach point F for the 3-8 combination, but there happens to be a good alternative. Make the 2 and draw the cueball to G. Carom the cueball lightly off the left side of the 3, pocketing the 8 and leaving yourself a good shot on the 3 into the corner pocket, Y. Follow the 3 to point F. Make the 4 in pocket W, following to point H. Make the 5, following to the side rail beyond the side pocket and rebounding to the vicinity of K. Pocket the 6 in the corner, and with deadball draw send the cueball a few inches past the side pocket. Make the 7 in the side and draw back to near the side pocket W for the 9.

If at any point in the run you lose position, consider laying down a safety. At the start, for example, if you come up short for position on the 2-ball—the cueball stopping near C—it would be easy to bank the 2 to C and leave the cueball behind the 4, 5, and 7.

As for riding the 9-ball in general, take that chance only when you are sure your opponent can't run out. Playing safe is almost always better than a wild shot.

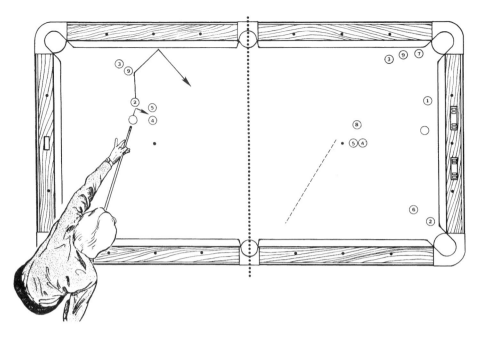

136 Caroms on offense and defense

Look at the right side of the diagram. How would you proceed? The 1 and 2 are easy, the 3 is in a bad spot. Even if you managed to bank the 3 somewhere, there is the 4-5 cluster to spread. A run-out is tough because of the location of the 7. A good player would see the solution at once. Pocket the 1 on a carom off the 7, bringing the 7 off the rail and clearing the way for the 3-9 combination. All you have to do then is make the 2 and get beyond the dashed line to have a shot at the 3, an easy game winner.

Keep your eyes peeled for easy carom shots to relocate inconvenient or interfering balls.

At the left is a partial layout of balls. You made the 1 but missed good position on the 2. An option to consider is caroming the 2-ball off the 9, sending the 2 uptable to the right and leaving the cueball snug against the 4 and the 5. If there are no other problems on the table, this shot makes you a big favorite to win the game. Other safeties can be played, but unless they break up the 9-3 cluster they are passive rather than aggressive because they don't improve your position.

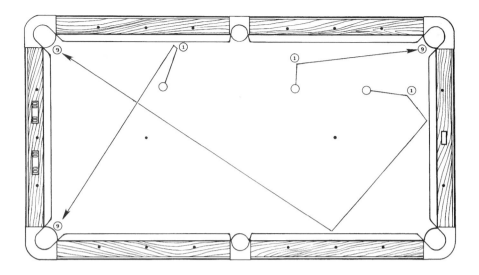

137 A game of sudden death

When the 9-ball ends up as part of an easy combination or is hanging in the jaws of a pocket, the character of the game instantly changes. Running out is no longer relevant; instead, the goal becomes getting a shot at the combo or making the 9 on a billiard (carom) shot.

Diagrammed are three easy billiard shots . . . easy, that is, if you are used to them. *They are well worth practicing* because variations of them come up frequently. You can think up additional patterns to work on. Shoot them over and over—changing the ball positions if you like—until you can at least come close to pocketing the 9 every time. Concentrating only on where the cueball is going instead of the object ball is not customary for pool players, so practice is required. It's hard to think of a practice drill for a student of nine-ball that pays off more generously.

If running the table is difficult, it can pay to play position for billiard shots like those in the diagram, especially if you'll be safe should you miss.

Danger! Control the speed carefully and land softly on the 9. Many beautiful billiard shots end in tragedy when the cueball follows the 9 into the pocket.

Finally, if the 9 is hanging or is part of a dead combination and you can hit the lowest-numbered ball only with a chancy bank, your best move might be to destroy the combo or pocket the 9 directly, even though it means giving your opponent ball in hand.

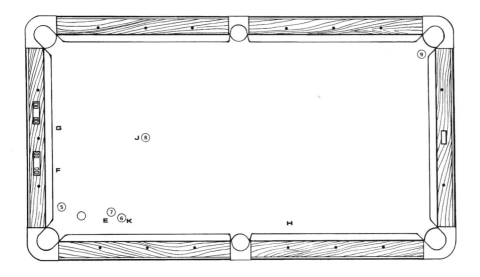

138 A game of inches and options

Sometimes the best choice of shot depends on the exact placement of the balls. An inch or even a fraction of an inch can make all the difference. In the diagram, the 9 is in front of the upper right pocket. There are a lot of possibilities to weigh. Banking the 5 into the 9 is a good bet, but be sure to shoot hard enough so that the 5 gets away from the 9 if you miss. Further protection is provided by the 6-7 cluster. When banking the 5, use either draw or follow with slight left to send the cueball to E. If the 9 doesn't drop and the cueball lands at E, your opponent is seriously stuck.

If the 5 is an inch closer to the letter F, the bank may be impossible because of the double-kiss. Two shots suggest themselves. Hit the 5 very thin on the left side with right English to send the cueball diagonally across the length of the table into the 9. The leave will be OK if the 5 stops somewhere between F and G.

Another idea—if the bank isn't there—is to go thin off the right side of the 5, driving it to E and sending the cueball to the vicinity of H for a safety.

What would you do if the cueball was stuck against the 6 at K instead of being in the diagrammed location? Very hard to make contact with the 5 from there. Consider pocketing the 9 and giving your opponent ball in hand. Because the 8 is on the spot, the 9 is placed frozen to it at J. A run-out is unlikely with two clusters to break, so you will at least get another turn.

What should your opponent do if you pocket the 9? Maybe put the cueball at F, make the 5, leave the cueball at E, and then shoot a stop shot on the 6, banking it to the center of the table while hooking you behind the 7. More aggressive players would break the 6 and 7 apart when making the 5, confident that they will be able to break the 8-9 cluster apart on one of their next two shots.

Pro players see the options in a matter of seconds and make accurate assessments of the odds of success on each one.

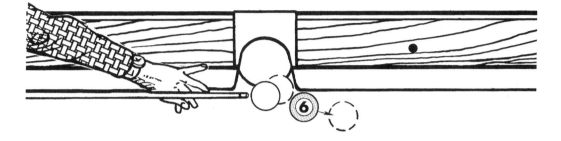

139 A dirty little safety

You have ball in hand. The 6 is on the rail close to the side pocket, but not so close that it can be made there. Is a run-out difficult? Is your loathsome opponent on two fouls? Fortunately for you, a sadistic safety beckons in this special situation. Put the cueball in the middle of the side pocket as shown, bump the 6 a few inches down the rail, and leave the cueball in the position of the dashed circle. Your opponent is corner hooked! Pretty hard for him or possibly her to both hit the 6 and leave you safe.

Reference: The shot is demonstrated on Pat Fleming's *The Creative Edge,* available from Accu-Stats Video Productions.

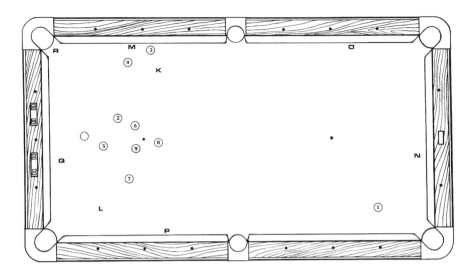

140 The treacherous push-out shot

If the first player breaks the balls, makes one or more balls, and doesn't like his leave, he is free to "push out," that is, simply knock the cueball anywhere. The second player can accept the position or force the breaker to shoot again. If nothing drops on the break, then the second player has the same option. The rule creates an interesting psychological face-off because the pusher offers his opponent a shot he is willing to take himself. Evenly matched players can't gain an advantage by pushing out; the best the pusher can hope for is to avoid a disadvantage.

Let's say you are hooked after the break and must push out. If the balls are spread and relatively easy to run, don't leave an open shot . . . or leave an open shot with the wrong angle for position. If it's a tough table to run, leaving an open shot is usually acceptable. The trap to avoid at all costs is giving your opponent a way to lay down a deadly safety.

In the diagram, pushing out to the upper rail near K is OK because even though the 1 is easy to make, the shot doesn't lead anywhere. Pushing out to the lower rail near L is a poor choice, in my opinion, because it is too easy to play safe off the left side of the 1, sending the cueball to N, O, P, and Q and leaving the 1-ball near N.

In some cases it is necessary to create a cluster to block a run-out—for example, by hitting the 4 softly to M to block the 3. Pocketing a ball is another option. In the diagram, if the 9 is hanging in the upper left pocket (R), better sink it. (The 9 is the only ball that respots when pocketed on a push-out.)

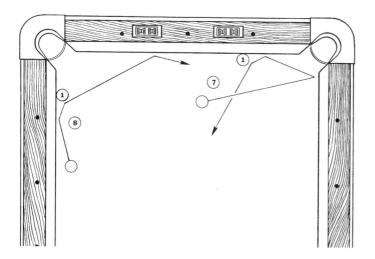

141 It can pay not to be so pushy

The danger of pushing out when hooked after the break is that your opponent will come to the table and make a winning shot, or do something nasty that you overlooked, thus covering you with ignominy in front of your loved ones, if any. If an easy rail-first hit is there, take it instead of pushing out and giving your opponent options. I wouldn't push out in either of the diagrammed positions—unless other balls blocked the cueball path after the hit. In both cases the hit is easy and the cueball can be sent to the other end of the table. Practice these two patterns a few times to learn how not to scratch in the side.

Warning! When deciding on a push-out, you must announce your intention. Otherwise, unless you drive a ball to a rail, you are guilty of a foul and your opponent can put the cueball anywhere.

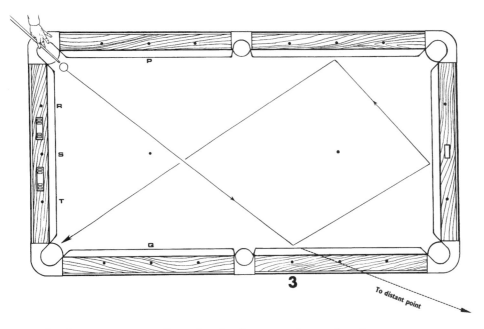

142 A kicking system for the judgment-impaired

When good nine-ball players are hooked and have to kick one or more rails to escape, they rely on judgment, not systems borrowed from the three-cushion world. If, however, you need help on multiple-rail banks, you might be interested in the "opposite three" system, designed to facilitate hitting any given point *on the fourth rail.*

If the cueball in the diagram is shot with running English so it contacts the nose of the first rail at a point opposite the third diamond, it will bank three rails and go into the lower left pocket, which is symmetrically opposite the starting point. A cueball starting at R, a diamond away from the corner, will return to T, a diamond away from the other corner. Start from P, return to Q. Note the symmetry between the starting point and the ending point. Shoot from S, equidistant from the two corners, and the cueball will return to the same point. In all cases, aim so that the cueball hits the first rail directly opposite the third diamond and use running English (left in the examples).

To handle less-than-ideal positions, use the "distant-point" technique familiar to three-cushion players. Let's say that the cueball is at R and the ball you have to hit is at S. If an around-the-table bank is the best option, the first step is to imagine where the cueball would have to be to make it an easy "opposite three" bank. In the example, it would be at S. Project an imaginary line from S through the point opposite three (the dashed line in the diagram) to a point roughly ten feet beyond the table. Mark the point in your mind's eye—it could be on the floor, on a wall, or on another table. Step back to the cueball and aim it at the distant point with running English. The cueball will return to S, or close to it.

Some experimenting with speed and English will be necessary to make the system work on your table and to learn what paths lead to the side pocket instead of to the fourth rail.

Reference: A fuller explanation of the opposite three system is given in *Byrne's Wonderful World,* Part Three. An end-rail-first system that can be applied to pool is explained in *Byrne's Advanced Technique*—see Diagrams 135 and 136.

How to win at nine-ball—a checklist

1. Develop an effective break. Use a stiff cue lighter or no heavier than your regular cue and with a thin, hard tip. Lengthen your bridge for a longer backswing. Concentrate on hitting the cueball a hair below center and the 1-ball full in the face. Read Twenty Keys to a Killer Break in *Byrne's Advanced Technique.*

2. When pushing out after the break, leave a low-percentage shot if the balls are spread and a 50-50 shot if they are clustered. Guard especially against giving the incoming player a way to bury the cueball.

3. If you are hooked with little chance of hitting the low ball—or of avoiding a sellout if you do hit it—consider creating a problem cluster.

4. Make sure you know the local rules! In the waning years of the twentieth century, the major nine-ball tournament associations have switched to all-balls-stay-down rules, presumably to speed up the game (it's already too fast) for television. Even balls made on scratches stay down, as do balls that land on the floor. Gone are the clever moves involving the spotting of illegally pocketed balls.

5. If a cluster prevents a run-out, watch for a chance to play a safety and at the same time spread the cluster. Accomplish that and you are suddenly a favorite to win the game. Read Double-Duty Defense in *Byrne's Wonderful World.*

6. When practicing, spend some time on safeties. Laying down a good hook requires closely controlling the blend of speed, spin, and hit . . . especially speed. Safety play is vitally important under prevailing rules and deserves practice. A good manager can beat a good shotmaker.

7. Practice escaping from safeties, too. You'll be glad you did.

8. Do you want to win or do you want to show off? If you want to win, don't go for the tough, sellout, sucker shots when there are safeties to be played.

9. Study top nine-ball players in tournaments or on tapes. You can't match their shotmaking, but you can learn a lot about position and safety.

10. Tournament winners are usually good at curving and jumping the cueball, techniques that can't be learned properly from a book, not even a book as deeply moving as this one. Take some lessons from a pro.

13

safeties, key balls, and break shots in straight pool

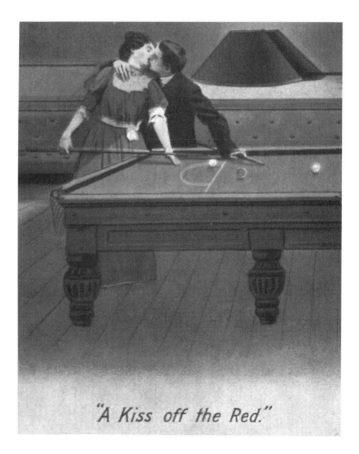

"A Kiss off the Red."

Postcard—1911
(Byrne Collection)

The championship game

A few decades ago, before eight-ball and nine-ball took over the tournament world, straight pool—or, as industry flacks would have it, 14.1 continuous pocket billiards—was called the championship game. The world pool champion was the player who won the national straight pool tournament. ("World" was the same as "national" because in those days the game was not well known outside the United States.) It's perhaps the most satisfying game to play or practice, maybe because even beginners can make a lot more balls than they miss.

In straight pool, you can make any ball at any time and each one counts one point. You must call the ball and the pocket. The winner is the player who reaches an agreed-upon number of points first, say 50 or 100. When the fourteenth ball is pocketed, those fourteen are racked and the last ball is left in place. If the shooter can break the pack while pocketing the loose ball, his run continues. Among the elite, runs of 100 are not uncommon.

The game requires delicacy, precision, and long-range planning. Unlike nine-ball and eight-ball, straight pool doesn't begin with a mindless gorilla break. Control, not raw power, is paramount.

There are several ways to level the playing field in matches between players of unequal strength. The stronger player can make at least five or ten shots in a row before he can count any, or he must bank his first shot, or he must make a greater number of points to win. The game is great for solo practice. It's fun to try to beat your high run.

Section 9 dealt with the analysis of the large clusters common in straight pool. Here we will deal with safety play, key balls, and break shots, subjects that are well understood by every competitive player.

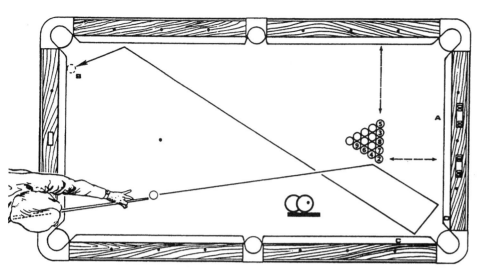

143 Safety play in straight pool—I

More games are lost by faulty defense than this world dreams of. It may be, in fact, that more games are lost than won, by which I mean that one player foolishly tries an extremely difficult shot, breaking the balls open for his opponent, or loses his patience during an exchange of deliberate safeties, leaving an open ball. Not trying to score, choosing instead to leave your opponent without a decent shot, is considered boring in some circles, even chicken. Yet it can be argued that good safety play requires more imagination, concentration, patience, and steely nerves— more skill, in a word—than shotmaking and positioning. Defensive skill is absolutely vital. When the Roman historian Tacitus (first name Cornelius) wrote in the year A.D. 110 that the desire for safety stands against every great and noble enterprise, he couldn't have been thinking of straight pool.

On the first shot of the game, diagrammed, two balls must be driven to a rail along with the cueball. The best way to do that without selling out is to clip the corner ball with right English, sending the cueball off three rails to B. In theory, the 2-ball will hit the end rail softly and the 5-ball will hit the side rail hard enough to return to the pack. Even if a ball or two become separated from the rest, the second player will have six or eight feet of green to traverse if he tries to score.

Once the game is under way, a safety is legal if only one ball touches a rail after the cueball contacts a ball, and that one ball can be the cueball. What should the second player do if the opening shot was executed perfectly? Safest is to lag the cueball softly from B to A to the rear of the pack. That costs one point, but against a good player it's better than taking the chance of leaving a makable shot by hitting the pack hard enough to drive a ball to the rail. Against a poor player, of course, you can shoot from a stepladder and still win.

Another possibility is to shoot from B to C. Done right, the cueball will hit D, lightly graze the 2, 4, 6, or 9, and return to B without significantly disturbing the balls.

If there are spaces between the balls in the 5-3-8-7-2 line and the cueball is at B, it is feasible to feather the left edge of the 5 and return to the left end rail. That won't work if the balls are frozen because the 2 will pop into the open.

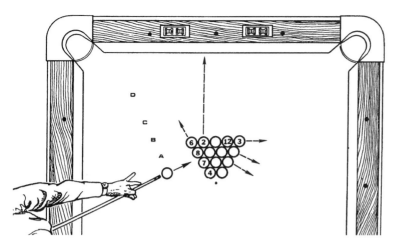

144 Safety play in straight pool—II

When you can't put a ball in a hole you might as well put your opponent there, which you can do from this position. Hit the right side of the 8 just hard enough to make the 2-ball reach the end rail. Several balls will pop out of the right side of the rack, and if you've left the cueball against the 8 and the 7, your opponent is in trouble. Make sure you don't bring the 2-ball off the end rail and back to the pack, because then the enemy can simply feather the 8 and leave you near the left corner pocket. Without that option he can only try to skim the 7 and leave the cueball at the far end of the table, hoping that you will miss the ensuing long shot.

Or he can test your knowledge of the game by placing his tip against the cueball and shoving it between the 8 and the 7. Such a stroke is illegal, but the only penalty is the loss of a point. Don't try something foolhardy in return. Accept the loss of a point yourself by moving the cueball an inch or two. Such cat and mouse play can't continue for long because the penalty for three fouls in a row is the loss of *fifteen* points, and since he started it he will be up against the wall first. In national-class competition, players have been known to accept the loss of fifteen points to avoid leaving an open shot.

From point A, hit the right side of the 6 just hard enough to send it to the end rail. From B, tickle the 4 and leave the cueball at the opposite end of the table, or hit the 6 squarely and leave the 3 on the rail. From C or D, feather the 4 or hit the 3 with left English, go to the side rail and the end rail, and come to rest near the starting point.

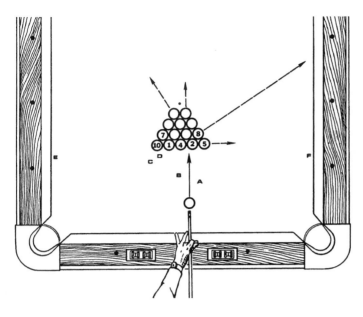

145 Safety play in straight pool—III

There are several safeties from the rear of the pack that partly spread the balls without leaving a makable shot. In the diagram, hit the left side of the 2, sending the 8 to the side rail and leaving the cueball against the 2 and the 4. From A, hit the left side of the 5 and send it to the rail. From B, hit the 2 squarely with stop-shot action, sending the 8 to the rail, or hit the 1 and send the 7 to the rail. Don't shoot so hard that the 5 or the 10 rebound off the side rails to knock the cueball away from a safe position.

From C, provided there are no balls elsewhere, barely hit the left side of the 10 and leave the cueball at the far end of the table. From D, go off the 10 to the side rail at E or off the 1 to the other side rail at F and back to a safe haven behind the pack.

In general, safety shots from the rear of the pack aren't as fruitful as those from the side because it is too easy for your opponent to return the favor by shooting off a ball to the side rail. Safeties into the side of the rack are more difficult to respond to. Best of all is leaving the cueball on the nameplate.

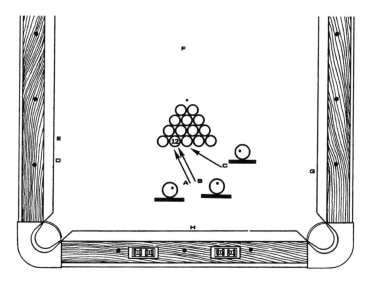

146 The break shot in straight pool—I

The choice of speed and English on a break shot often depends on the angle of approach and the point of contact. Above, a cueball moving along line A will hit the left side of the 12-ball and will either push through the corner ball or carom to the side rail near E. Right English should be used as well as follow so that the cueball, if it hits the rail, will rebound to the vicinity of F. On line B, the cueball will hit the 12 squarely and will not carom to the left. Use straight follow with enough power to make the cueball push forward a foot or two.

From a shallow angle like C, there is no chance that the cueball will push through the balls . . . it will carom off the rack to the side rail near D. Use left English to send the cueball from D to H, to G, and, ideally, to F.

On all break shots, try to keep the cueball from drifting beyond the center of the table.

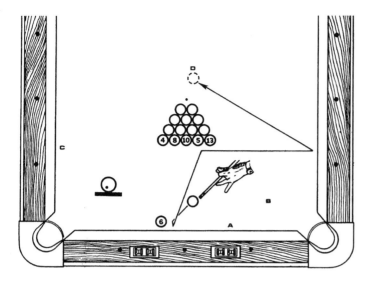

147 The break shot in straight pool—II

When bouncing off a rail into the rack, the danger is that the cueball will be left stuck to one of the almost immovable central balls, like the 10 in the diagram. To guard against that, go for the balls in the corners when you can, which are free to roll clear, and try to approach them at an angle so that the cueball will carom away from the pack. Above, low left will bring the cueball into the 5 and 13, then to the side rail and out to D. If the object ball and the cueball were a diamond to the right to begin with, at points A and B, then right English should be used to send the cueball into the 8 and 4, to point C, and to D.

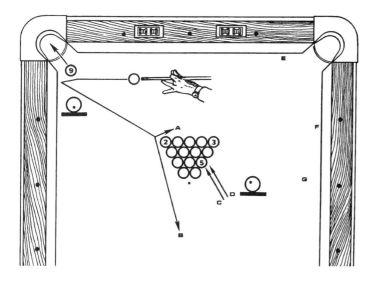

148 The break shot in straight pool—III

A cueball on the C line will hit the 5-ball squarely. Follow and a fairly hard stroke are needed to make sure the cueball doesn't stick to the side of the rack. On line D the cueball will carom to the right. To make sure the cueball doesn't roll to the far end of the table, use left English to kill the speed when it touches the rails at E and F. The goal is to stop at G.

The break off the 9 is risky, and there is some disagreement among experts on how best to handle it. One approach is to use a soft stroke and carom off the 2 to B or a foot or so beyond, trusting that the 3 at least will be separated from the rack. Most players shoot fairly hard and try to hit the 2 squarely, even though the cueball might scratch along line A or roll to the far end along line B.

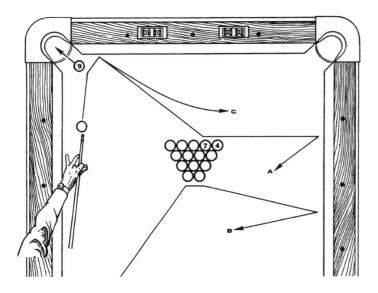

149 The break shot in straight pool—IV

When cutting a ball into the corner pocket from this position, try to carom into the 7-ball, then to the side rail and out to A or a foot or two beyond. Don't hit the cueball high or you are liable to see your hopes evaporate along the curved path C.

The best place to hit the pack from a side-pocket break ball is between the two head balls. Use a touch of high English to make sure the cueball doesn't scratch in the side along line B.

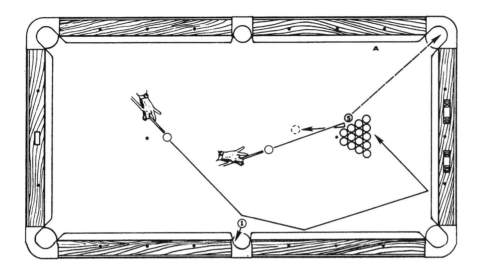

150 The break shot in straight pool—V

Don't overlook the possibility of getting the cueball away from the rack with draw. From the given position, follow might send the cueball into the corner pocket along with the 5-ball, or off two rails to the left end of the table. Draw is a good bet here. If the cueball can be brought back as shown, there will almost certainly be a shot into the lower right-hand corner pocket.

The cueball at the left could be drawn directly off the 1-ball into the rack, but without much zip. The rack can be hit harder with a two-rail bank as shown. Go for the far corner of the triangle, carom to A and out to the area around the dashed ball.

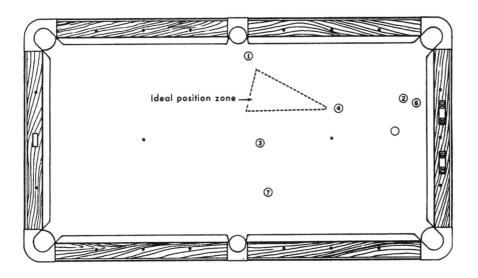

Ideal position zone →

151 Key balls and break balls

High runs depend on being able to break the pack off the fifteenth ball after the first fourteen are racked. Once the pack is broken, the idea is to pick out a ball or two that would make good break balls as well as key for playing position on them. Try to leave those balls undisturbed while pocketing the rest.

In the diagram, the 4-ball is a perfect break ball, provided the cueball can be left in the outlined position zone. The zone can most easily be reached off the 1, so the 1 is the key ball. A possible sequence: 2 in the corner, draw straight back one foot; 6 in the corner, rebound several inches past the 4; 3 in the side, follow one foot; 7 in the corner, stop the cueball; 1 in the side, rebound softly into the position zone.

If, after the 6, the position on the 3 is not so hot, leave it as the key ball and make the 1 and 7 first. Some players get into trouble by becoming emotionally attached to their first plan.

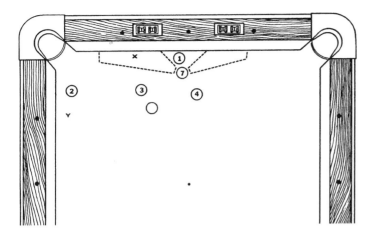

152 More on break balls and key balls

The game is straight pool and five balls are left. The 7 would provide a good break from either of the outlined position zones. What sequence of shots would you adopt? What is the key ball? Decide before reading the answer.

Shoot a stop shot on the 4. Use follow on the 3, sending the cueball to point Y. Pocket the 2 with follow, landing at X. Now either follow or draw off the 1, whichever seems easiest.

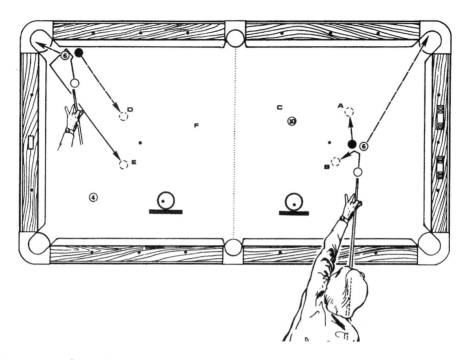

153 "Manufacturing" the break ball

Sometimes an apparently useless ball can be transformed into a break ball by bumping it to a new position. Two examples are shown. At the right, the black ball can be sent to A when the 6 is pocketed. A little draw puts the cueball at B. Now the 10 can be made in the side, and by allowing the cueball to roll forward to C, the player has left himself a perfect break shot. The tactic is called "manufacturing" a break ball.

The secret of the position at the left involves a use of English that is helpful on many kinds of shots. Hit the cueball on the left side and cut the 6 in the corner. The cueball will carom off the black ball and two rails and stop, if the speed is right, at or near E. The black ball will roll to D. From E it is no problem to make the 4 and draw the cueball to the neighborhood of F, just right for a break off the black ball.

Reference: For more on straight pool, see *Winning Pocket Billiards,* by Willie Mosconi, and *Advanced Pool,* by George Fels (Contemporary Books, Chicago, 1995).

14

favorite trick shots

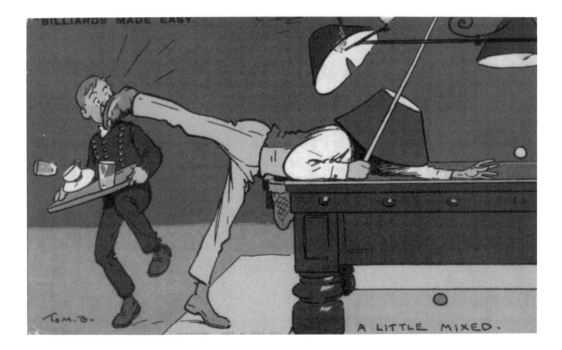

Postcard—1906
(Byrne Collection)

Having fun with trick shots

There are so many trick shots, with more being concocted all the time, that some-body should write a book about them—so I did. *Byrne's Treasury of Trick Shots,* published by Harcourt Brace in 1982, features descriptions of some 300 special shots that can be called trick, skill, fancy, stroke, novelty, or artistic. One of my goals was to supply historical background and uncover as many origins and in-ventors as possible. A revolutionary concept at the time was the effort to give credit where credit was due.

I noted that many of the shots in the repertories of today's exhibition players can be traced back to such works as *Le Noble Jeu de Billard,* by Captain François Mingaud (Paris, 1827), *The McCleery Method of Billiard Playing,* by J. F. B. Mc-Cleery (San Francisco, 1890), *Championship Billiards Old and New,* by John Thatcher (Chicago, 1898), *Fun on the Pool Table,* by Fred Herrmann (New York, 1902), *Trick and Fancy Pool Shots Exposed,* by Joseph Godfrey Hood (Roxbury, Mas-sachusetts, 1908), and *Trick and Fancy Shots in Pocket Billiards Made Easy,* by Jimmy Caras (Springfield, Pennsylvania, 1948). The books by Hood (an especially rich source) and Herrmann are the first ever published on the modern game of pool (as opposed to caroms or games played on tables with rounded pocket openings).

Creative players have come up with hundreds of new shots since my 1982 treatise, and the juices continue to flow. I included chapters on new and unusual shots in *Byrne's Advanced Technique* (1990) and *Byrne's Wonderful World* (1996).

It's unhealthy to work on improving solely to make other people feel bad by beating them in games. Forget competition and rules once in a while and have some fun with trick shots. The sampling of old favorites and new arrivals in the following pages, none of them requiring unusual gifts, is intended to persuade the overly serious to relax a little and enjoy life.

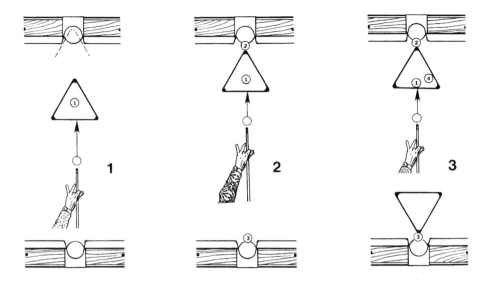

154 Evolution of the triangle slide

Place a 1-ball, a triangle, and a cueball on the table as shown in shot 1, left, and challenge a friend to make the 1. Looks impossible, but in fact couldn't be easier. Simply shoot straight ahead and force the triangle to slide across the table until its apex is in the side pocket (dashed lines). The 1-ball will be herded forward until it drops. Hood diagrammed the shot in 1908.

In the 1970s and maybe earlier, somebody thought of adding a couple of more balls, as in shot 2, above. Backspin on the cueball will draw it back to make the 3.

On Easter Sunday 1997, Ward Scott of Houston, Texas, was showing the shot to his five-year-old niece, Lauren, who placed a 4-ball inside the rack as shown at the right (shot 3). Ward found after a little experimenting with the positions, all four balls can be made. Call this latest version Lauren's Shot.

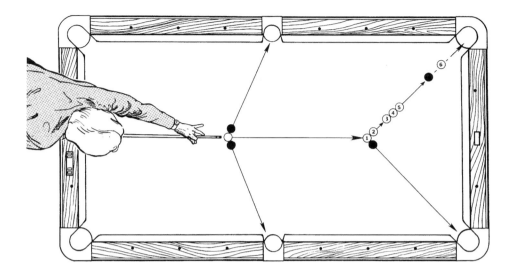

155 The "Little French Airplane" shot

The diagram is patterned after a shot sent to me by Eric Dubois of Toulouse, France. The challenge is to make only the four black balls. It can't be done without resting the upper right black ball on a piece of chalk. When the 5-ball hits it, the final black ball will jump all the way over the 6-ball and into the pocket, possibly on the fly. You'll have to shoot it a few times to discover the proper speed.

When setting it up, use your cue to align the 1, 2, 3, 4, 5, black, and 6 balls. A three-ball combination is used to make sure the 5-ball isn't thrown off line and hits the black ball squarely. The gaps in the line of balls create an amusing delayed reaction.

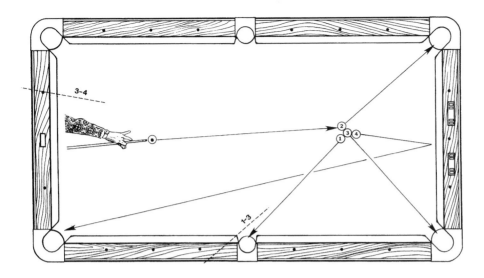

156 John Delaveau's "Guess Where" shot

Put the 1-ball on the foot spot, the cueball on the head spot, and the other three balls as diagrammed. The dashed lines show how to line up the 3-4 and the 1-3 combinations. The 2-3 combo is aimed straight at the center of the corner pocket. A solid hit on the 2 will send all balls into pockets, though the bank of the 4 is not a certainty.

    Delaveau always presents the shot as a challenge. Where will the four balls go? For some reason, onlookers seldom predict the path of the 3.

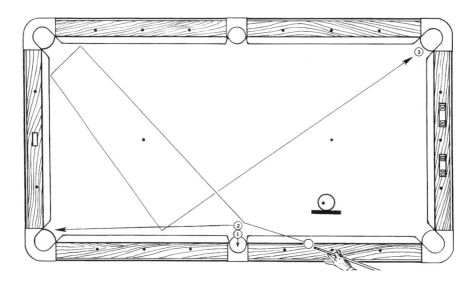

157 Around the world with Ivor Bransford

If the shot is not too hard, you can sometimes add a bit of showmanship by start-ing with the cueball on top of the rail. (If the cueball won't stay put, rest it against a piece of chalk.)

Diagrammed is a shot I learned from Ivor Bransford in 1980. It can be set up in an instant and made at least half the time even on a table you've never seen before. It's one of those shots beloved by exhibition players that is easier than it looks. Stroke it with authority.

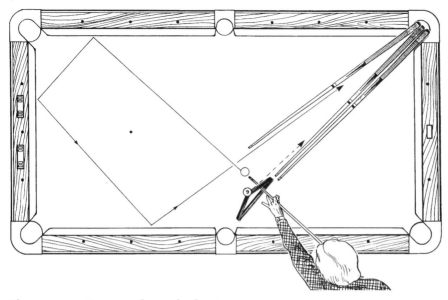

158 The repeating railroad shot

It's not true that there is nothing new under the sun. Rick Wright took the old railroad theme and added something never seen before. In a program of trick shots, this might be the one the flabbergasted audience remembers. You'll need a table big enough to accept three cues and a triangle as shown. Put an indentation on one corner of the triangle big enough to hold a ball.

Arrange the cues in the customary railroad position, place the triangle upright, and balance a 9-ball on top. Note the exact alignment of the triangle. You can begin in several ways; I show the player shooting through the triangle.

Here's what happens if all goes well. The cueball, struck with running English, banks off three rails, climbs the cues, turns the corner around the rim of the pocket, rolls down the other pair of cues, and bumps into the edge of the triangle, nudging it a little to the left. The 9 is dislodged from its perch, rolls down the side of the triangle, *and repeats the cueball's path up and down the cues!* If the triangle was located exactly right to begin with, the 9 will roll into the side pocket. What an idea!

If the 9 lacks the speed to climb the cues, Rick suggests propping up the right corner of the triangle with a matchbox; with a ramp that isn't quite so steep, less cueball energy is lost in bouncing on the cloth.

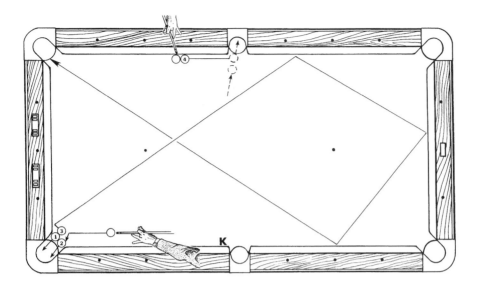

159 Charlie Webster's shot . . . and more

Two personal favorites, one well known, one not. Consider the balls in the lower left corner. Can they all be made in one shot? Charlie Webster found a way in a game of one-pocket in which he needed to make a ball in the upper left corner to win. When trying the diagrammed pattern, aim the 1-3 combination directly at the center of the opposite side pocket. Use slight left on the cueball and hit half the 3-ball. If the 3 fails to drop, make the necessary adjustment to the 1-3 combo line.

At the top is the timed bank that has been a favorite since Joe Hood included it in his 1908 book. The cueball and the 4 are frozen to each other and to the rail. Aim the cueball at point K—an inch or two from the edge of the side pocket— with just enough left sidespin to bring it back to the side. Pick point K properly and the 4 will move along the rail just far enough to get knocked into the side pocket.

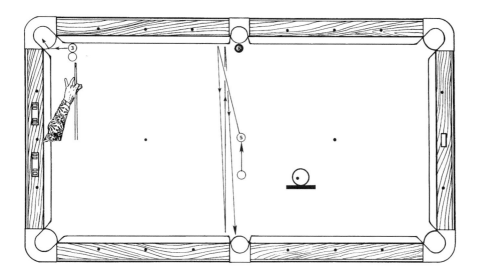

160 The triple bank and the push squeeze

Paul Gerni showed me how to triple bank a ball from the center of the table just in time to include it in my 1982 *Treasury*. I present it now as a sensational way to end a game of eight-ball. The 5 is on the center spot and the 8 is blocking the side. What should be done? It looks like the only option is a very tough bank in the corner. But wait! Bring the audience to its feet cheering with a triple bank in the side! Use heavy left sidespin and try not to smile when it goes. It's another example that bank shots aren't simple exercises in plane geometry.

At the upper left is a shot you can teach to your tiny daughter when she gets home from soccer practice. The 3 can be squeezed into the corner pocket by placing the cue tip against the right side of the cueball and pushing, not stroking. Leave us not mention the illegality.

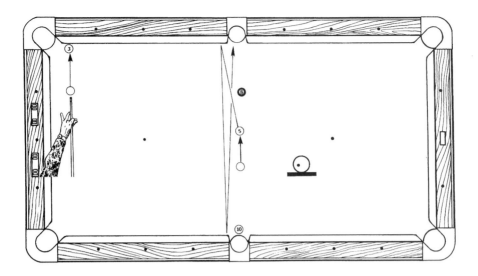

161 Two old friends of mine you may have met

Not only can a ball on the center spot be triple banked, it can be double banked as well if you catch it just right. I use a gamelike situation to present it to stunned onlookers. It's your shot in a game of eight-ball and the 5 is your last ball. The 8 blocks the straight-in shot and the 10 rules out the triple bank. So double bank it as diagrammed.

At the upper left, the 3 is frozen to the rail. Can it be banked into the lower left corner? Yes, if you use a tennis ball instead of a cueball. The action is comical.

Reference: Several of the preceding shots in this section are demonstrated and shown from different camera angles on *Byrne's Standard Video of Trick Shots, Vols. III and IV.*

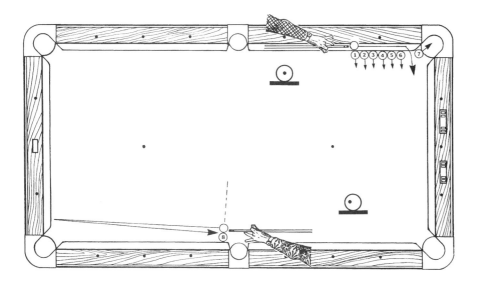

162 Two Swiss confections

Six balls are frozen to the rail and to each other as shown in the upper right-hand corner of the diagram. The 7-ball is hanging in the jaws. Hand the cueball to a friend and tell him he can put it anywhere. The challenge is to contact every ball with the cueball and also pocket the 7-ball. The only way to do it is to place the cueball on top of the rail so it rests against the end ball. Shoot along the top of the rail just hard enough so that the cueball hits each ball in succession before falling to the table to pocket the 7.

At the bottom, the 8-ball is frozen to the rail a half-inch from the side pocket and the cueball is frozen to it. The two balls are angled slightly off perpendicular. The 8 can be made in the side by means of a time shot. Shoot parallel to the rail, which will bring the 8-ball an inch or so off the rail. The returning cueball, if the pool gods smile, will pocket the 8 in the side. You'll need a little left English.

These two ingenious shots are inventions of Sebastien Pauchon of Vevey, Switzerland. He sent me diagrams in 1997 because he knew I wouldn't show them to anybody. Turn the page for another of his brainstorms.

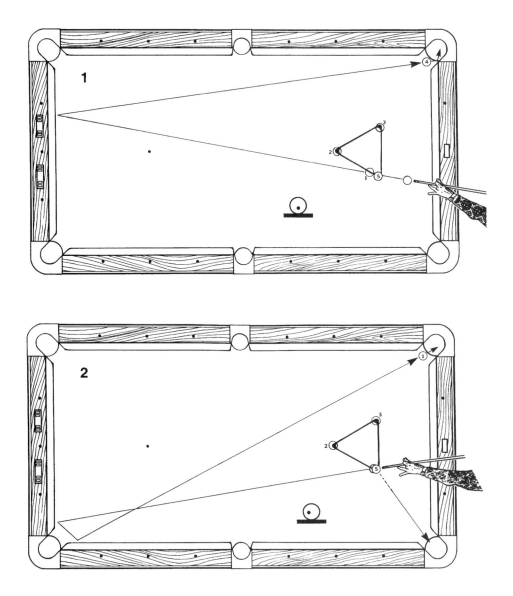

163 The double-stroke balancing act

Balance a triangle on the 1-, 2-, and 3-balls. (See top diagram.) Note how the 1-ball is offset. Atop the triangle place the 5-ball. (Dent the wood to keep it in position.) Using stop-shot action, bank the 1-ball softly into the 4. Do it right and the cueball replaces the 1-ball and the triangle doesn't fall. Now shoot the cueball with left English so it banks two rails to pocket the 1-ball (lower diagram). Withdraw your cue quickly to avoid the falling triangle and watch the 5-ball roll into the corner. Nice shot, Sebastien!

collecting billiard memorabilia

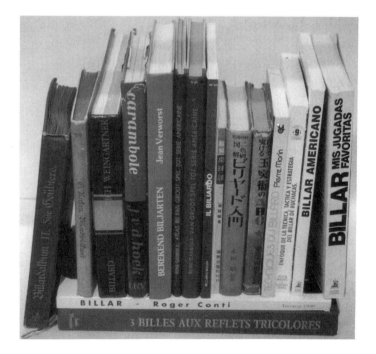

Billiard books in German, Dutch, Italian, Chinese, Japanese, French, and Spanish.
(Byrne Collection)

The world of Billiardiana

A striking change since the first version of this book appeared in 1978 is the increased interest in the game's history, books, graphics, art, furniture, signage, artifacts, iconography, photography, ephemera, effluvia, and detritus. Rarely anymore can you get anything worth collecting for a song. When I started accumulating odds and ends in the early 1960s, the game was in one of its periodic lulls and you could find all sorts of neat stuff in secondhand bookstores, antique shops, and even junk piles. Old billiard postcards and magazines with relevant articles or photos could be bought for a few dimes and early books for a few dollars. There was no organized secondary market and the buying was easy.

Not so today! A decades-long boom in cue games worldwide has spawned a legion of hunter-gatherers. Billiard postcards from the turn of the century now are worth between five and twenty dollars and books published a hundred to a hundred and fifty years ago can fetch a thousand. Telephone auctions of billiard-related materials are held twice a year by New Deco, Inc., of Boca Raton, Florida, and generate a lot of action.

I have dipped often into my own collection to illustrate my pool and billiard books, especially this one. In the following pages are further examples in a variety of categories.

For more information on a vast and fascinating world, see the auction catalogs published by New Deco (800-543-3326) and the chapter The Pleasures of Collecting in *Byrne's Wonderful World.*

For reproductions in full color, see:

Pool, by Mike Shamos, Mallard Press, New York, 1991;

The Illustrated Encyclopedia of Billiards, by Mike Shamos, Lyons & Burford, New York, 1993; and

The Billiard Encyclopedia, by Victor Stein and Paul Rubino, second edition, Blue Book Publications, Minneapolis, Minnesota, 1996.

Magazines

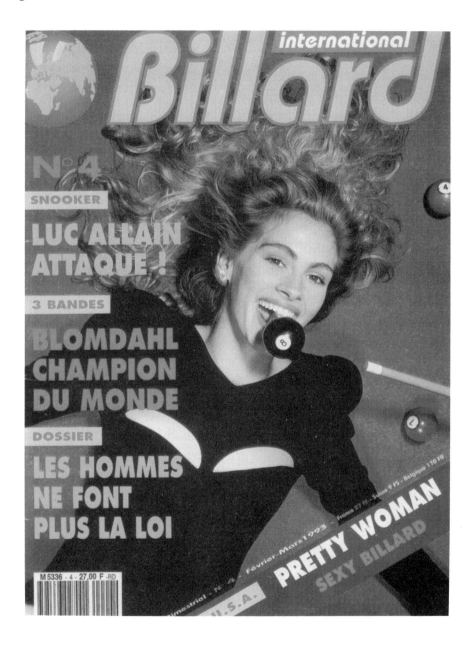

Putting her famous smile to good use, Julia Roberts clamps a piece of chalk between her teeth to hold an 8-ball for the "shoot-off-the-mouth" shot. *Billard International,* the most colorful billiard monthly in the world, is published in Nogent sur Marne, France.

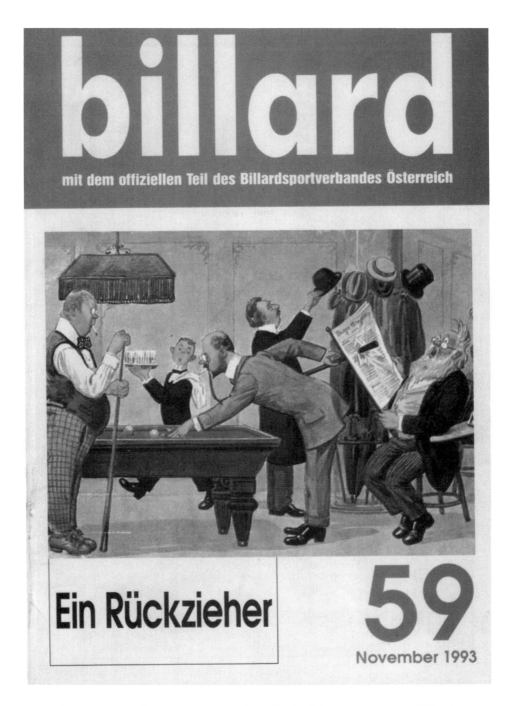

billard

mit dem offiziellen Teil des Billardsportverbandes Österreich

Ein Rückzieher

59

November 1993

Heinrich Weingartner of Vienna, Austria, editor of *Billard,* has put together a billiard museum, manufactures billiard tables, owns a popular billiard room/coffeehouse, and is a respected teacher and player. His magazine often features graphics from his extensive collection.

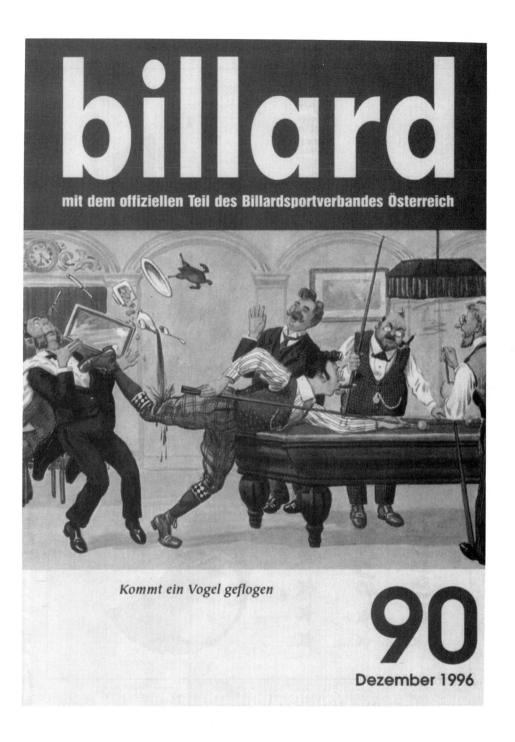

billard

mit dem offiziellen Teil des Billardsportverbandes Österreich

Kommt ein Vogel geflogen

90

Dezember 1996

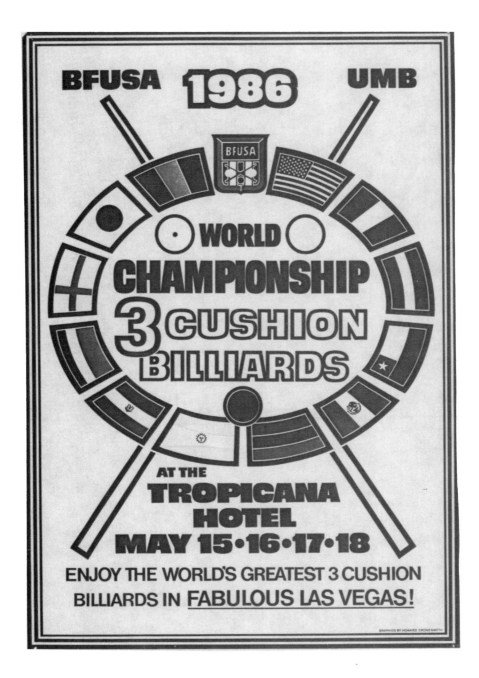

The late Howard Cronenweth of Los Angeles, a Disney artist, created an attractive poster for a billiard tournament in Las Vegas using a "flags-of-all-entrants" theme.

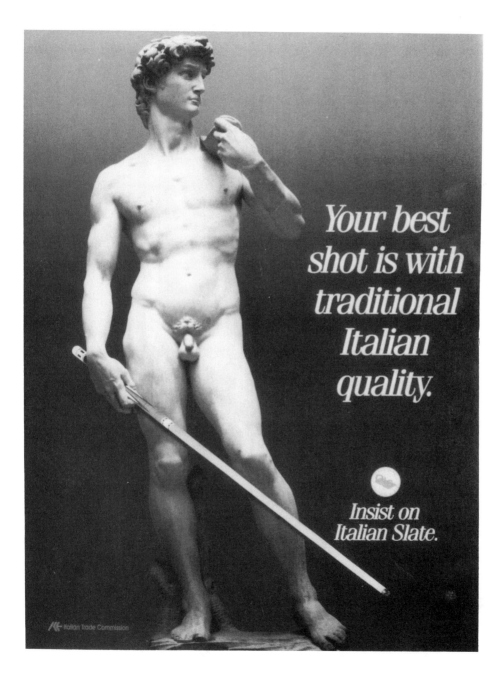

A poster distributed by the Italian Trade Commission in support of Italian table slate.

Novelties

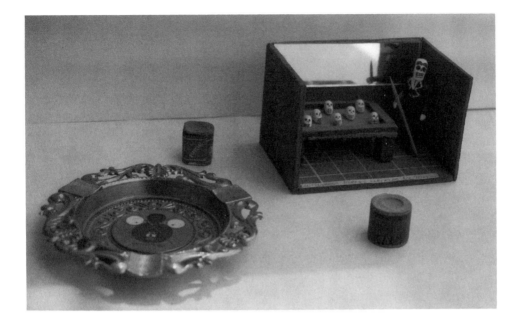

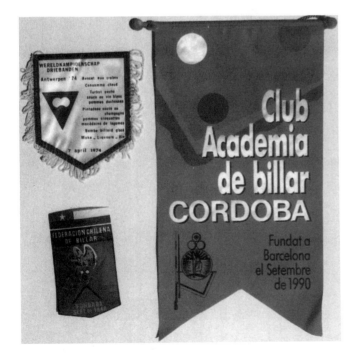

There are a lot of skulls, skeletons, and death in Mexican folk culture, as evidenced by the novelty above, right, bought from a street vendor in Mexico City. Also in the photo are two pieces of antique chalk and a souvenir ashtray from a billiard club in Villajoyosa, Spain. At left are small pennants from Spain, Belgium, and Chile.

Book jackets and illustrations

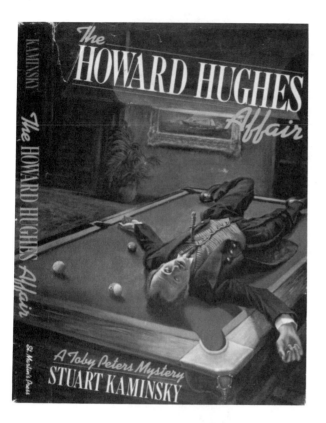

ABOVE: Housewives have used pool tables for centuries to fold laundry. Another use is depicted on the cover of *The Howard Hughes Affair*, a novel by Stuart Kaminsky published by St. Martin's Press in 1979, painting by Joel Iskowitz. Pool plays no part in the novel.

RIGHT: An illustration by Elaine Duillo from *The Wedding Gamble*, by Cait Logan, a romance published in paperback by Dell in 1996. The heroine is a glamorous pool hustler in the Montana of the old west.

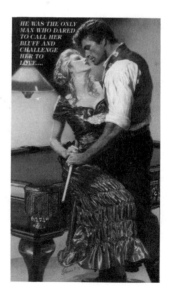

Player cards

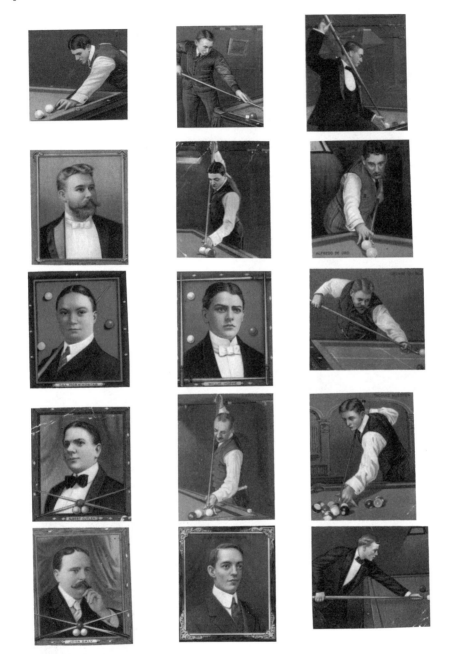

In the early years of the twentieth century, billiard cards were as popular as baseball cards. Mecca Cigarettes released a set of fifteen cards in about 1911 featuring the best-known pool and billiard champions.

Autographs

A handwritten letter from Willie Hoppe to Danny McGoorty. The letter reads: "Miami Beach, Oct. 11, 1957. Dear Danny: Your card came this morning. Thanks so much for remembering my birthday. Have been living here for a year and really like it. Of course, I go north about twice a year to beat this hot weather. Play once in a while—do a little teaching as do miss the game of billiards as it's been greater part of my life. Want to wish you lots of success in your club. If I get out there next spring will drop in to see you—plan to go out to see the children. Again thanking you for your kindness. Regards to all, and yourself. Willie Hoppe."

Souvenir photos

A happy scene at the trade show of the Billiard Congress of America, Louisville, Kentucky, July 23, 1988. Left to right are Jean Balukas, Robert Byrne, Dorothy Wise, Willie Mosconi, Jerry Briesath, and Irving Crane.

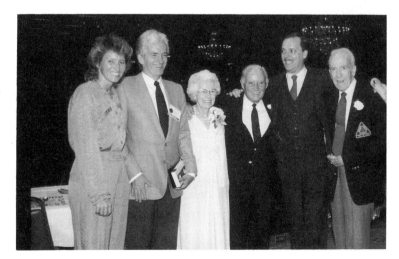

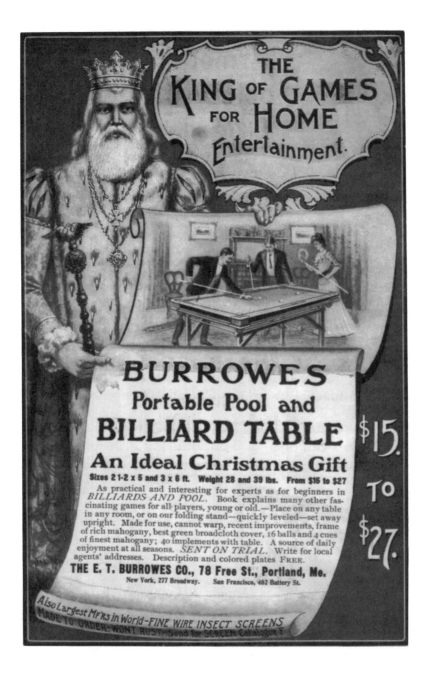

Early magazine ads are eminently collectible. I bought this one at a flea market.

Exhibition announcements

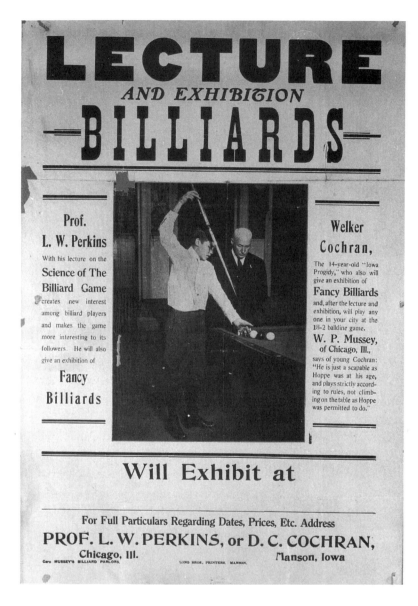

LECTURE
AND EXHIBITION
BILLIARDS

Prof. L. W. Perkins

With his lecture on the **Science of The Billiard Game** creates new interest among billiard players and makes the game more interesting to its followers. He will also give an exhibition of

Fancy Billiards

Welker Cochran,

The 14-year-old "Iowa Progidy," who also will give an exhibition of **Fancy Billiards** and, after the lecture and exhibition, will play any one in your city at the 18-2 balkline game.

W. P. Mussey, of Chicago, Ill., says of young Cochran: "He is just a scapable as Hoppe was at his age, and plays strictly according to rules, not climbing on the table as Hoppe was permitted to do."

Will Exhibit at

For Full Particulars Regarding Dates, Prices, Etc. Address

PROF. L. W. PERKINS, or D. C. COCHRAN,
Chicago, Ill. Manson, Iowa
Care MUSSEY'S BILLIARD PARLORS. LONG BROS. PRINTERS, MANSON.

In 1911, broadsides were printed to facilitate a tour of Midwest rooms by legendary teacher Lanson W. Perkins and his star pupil, Welker Cochran. Note the reference to another child prodigy, Willie Hoppe, who was nine years older than the new whiz kid.
(Byrne Collection)

Movie stills

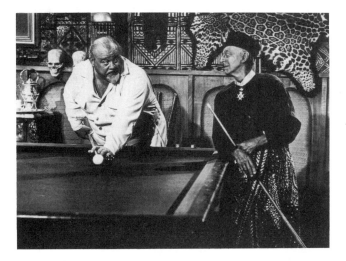

In the 1962 film *The Spiral Road* (RKO), set in Java during a leprosy epidemic, Burl Ives shows why it was lucky he could sing. Film critic Leslie Halliwell called the flick "a long slog through the jungle with a hilariously miscast star."

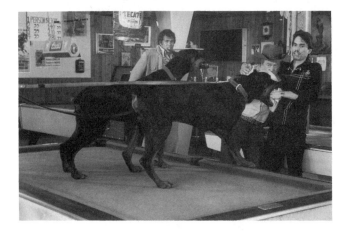

Rented attack dogs neutralize local toughs, enabling pool hustlers James Coburn and Bruce Boxleitner to escape with their lives. The scene was filmed but later cut from *The Baltimore Bullet* (Avco Embassy/Filmfair, 1980). The movie, a disappointment despite cameos by many pro players, is worth watching on video for the pool scenes. Omar Sharif is oddly unconvincing as a big-time money player, even though he was an excellent three-cushion player as a youth in Egypt.

16

rules of major pool games

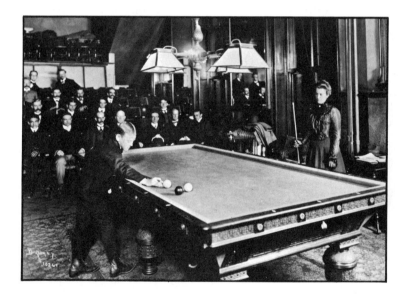

Willie Hoppe at twelve, with his mother.
(The Byron Collection, Museum of the City of New York)

Straight pool

Straight pool, also called rack pool and—by industry flacks—14.1 continuous pocket billiards, is one of three games used to measure skill at the highest level, the others being nine-ball and one-pocket. Eight-ball is an inadequate test.

Straight pool is a call-shot game. To score you must name a ball and the pocket you intend to put it in. You don't have to hit the called ball first and you don't have to describe by what means or route it will get to the pocket—to that extent, slop counts. Except for tournament play, however, players usually don't bother saying anything unless their intentions aren't obvious.

The numbers on the balls are used only to facilitate the calling of shots. Making a called ball counts one point, and the winner is the one who first reaches an agreed-upon total. If the called ball goes in, then other balls that drop on the same stroke also each count one point. Players shoot until they miss, commit a foul, or win the game.

At the start, fifteen balls are racked on the foot spot and the cueball is behind the head string. The player who opens must drive two balls and the cueball to a rail. Failure to do so is penalized by the loss of two points, giving the breaker a score of minus two. The second player then has the option of shooting or making the first player start over with the balls reracked and the same penalties and restrictions in force.

After the break, fouls cost one point. Three fouls in a row cost an additional fifteen points. It is a foul to touch a ball with hands, cue, or clothing, to hit the cueball twice on one stroke, to scratch, to jump the cueball off the table, to shoot while balls are moving or spinning, and to shoot without at least one foot on the floor. On every shot, you must either drive a ball to a rail, pocket a ball, or make the cueball hit a rail after hitting a ball; failure to do so is a foul.

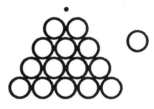

When only one object ball is left on the table, the rest are racked with the foot spot open, as shown in the diagrams in the nine-ball section. The player who made the fourteenth ball continues to shoot until he misses, as he almost certainly will soon if he doesn't make the fifteenth ball and break up the pack at the same time.

If the fifteenth ball interferes with the racking of the other fourteen, it is placed on the head spot. If the cueball interferes with the racking of the balls, the shooter has it in hand behind the head string. If they both interfere, all fifteen balls are racked in a triangle and the cueball is in hand behind the head string. If the cueball interferes with the rack and the fifteenth ball is behind the head string, the cueball is put on the head spot unless the fifteenth ball is already there, in which case the cueball goes on the exact center of the table.

A player may choose to play safe, in which case he must drive a ball to a rail or make the cueball hit a rail after hitting a ball. It is not a legal safety to shoot at a ball frozen to a rail unless the ball is pocketed, is driven to another rail, or the cueball touches a rail after hitting the ball. If a ball is within a ball-width of a rail, only two safeties can be played off it—on the third shot it is treated as a ball frozen to a rail.

If the called ball jumps the table, it is considered a miss and not a foul. The ball is placed on the foot spot or as near to it as possible along a line running from the foot spot to the center of the foot rail. If the called ball is made and another ball goes off the table, the jumped ball is spotted and the shooter's inning continues.

It is legal to play safe off a ball to which the cueball is frozen by regarding the balls as not frozen.

In deciding whether or not a ball is on one side of the head string or the other, consider only the spot where the ball touches the cloth.

A ball that bounces out of a pocket is judged never to have gone in.

Line-up straight pool

Identical to rack straight pool except for when and how pocketed balls return to play. In line-up, the balls are returned when the shooter misses. The incoming player, therefore, always begins with fifteen balls. The returned balls are spotted in a straight line behind the foot spot, with gaps as small as possible left in the line to clear interfering balls. If necessary, the line is continued in front of the foot spot. If a player runs fifteen balls in a row, they are lined up and the inning continues.

Equal Offense

A variation of straight pool is Equal Offense, copyrighted in 1976 by Jerry Briesath, owner of Cue-Nique Billiards and the beautiful new Green Room in Madison, Wisconsin. Two weaknesses of rack pool are eliminated: boring exchanges of deliberate safeties and the possibility of losing without getting a chance to score. Tournaments of Equal Offense are based on medal rather than match play.

General straight pool rules apply. Each player gets ten turns at the table, and he shoots until he misses, fouls, scratches, or runs twenty. The maximum possible score, therefore, is two hundred. At the beginning of each inning, the player breaks apart the rack of fifteen balls as fully as possible. On the break there is no penalty for scratching, and any balls that go in are respotted. The player has the cueball in hand behind the head string to begin shooting whether he scratched or not.

The score is kept on a sheet with ten frames, as in bowling, with enough room in each box to write the inning score along with the cumulative score. A nice feature of the game is that it is good for solo practice and for players who want to keep track of their progress. In a tournament, all players advance simultaneously, and with a large scoreboard the spectators can become enthralled with everybody's relative position.

It's a good game for players of unequal strength because it is so easy to handicap. The stronger player can be given fewer innings or a lower high-run limit. The weaker player can be given more than one miss per inning or can be allowed to place the cueball anywhere on the table after breaking the balls.

(Briesath passes along a suggestion for teachers of pool. Get beginners started early in thinking ahead and planning sequences of shots. To do it, spread the balls around the table and ask them to find a spot for the cueball that would result in three simple shots in a row. As a teacher, Briesath has produced half-a-dozen male and female intercollegiate champions and regularly travels to put on three-day clinics.)

Because Equal Offense is a relatively new game, one is tempted to tinker with the rules. My feeling is that it might be good to give some sort of bonus for running more than a few balls. The game could be scored like bowling, with a run of ten (or any agreed-upon total) counted as a spare and twenty counted as a strike. To minimize the amount of racking, try letting each player continue shooting until he has pocketed twenty balls, keeping track of misses. The player with the fewest misses at the end of an agreed-upon number of "frames" wins.

It would be wonderful if by this modification of Briesath's invention some of the allure of bowling is given to pool. I have long pondered bowling's popularity. It is based in part, I think, on knocking things down and making noise, but even more on the exhilarating bonuses built into the scoring system. Would we be groaning under so many bowlers if their scores were the simple sum of pins toppled? I think not.

Nine-ball

Gamblers like nine-ball because money changes hands quickly and spectators like it because the players frequently must try spectacular shots.

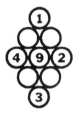

Only the nine lowest-numbered balls are used, and they are racked in a diamond shape with the 1 at the apex and the 9 buried in the middle. Anything that drops on the break counts if the 1 is hit first. Anything that drops on any subsequent shot counts if the cueball hits the lowest-numbered ball first. The game is won by the player who makes the 9 on a legal shot—thus the game can end on the break, on a combination, or when the 9 is pocketed as the last ball. Under the new rules, balls are never respotted—except for the 9.

Most nine-ball is now played with the "push-out" rule. If a player breaks, makes a ball, and leaves himself hooked—or if he fails to make a ball and leaves the second player hooked—the player at the table can announce a push shot. The cueball is simply rolled to a position that provides a clear shot at the low ball. The other player can either accept the position or force the pusher to shoot again. Pushing out is an option only after the break shot. Push-outs are not fouls only if they are announced.

The full-table ball-in-hand rule has almost entirely replaced the behind-the-line rule for punishing fouls. The penalty is so great it pays to watch for chances to play deliberate safeties.

One-pocket

Hustlers can win in one-pocket without making a single outstanding shot. The sucker never realizes what he is up against because knowledge, craftiness, and patience are as well-rewarded as shotmaking ability. Feeble old men can beat hotshots by outmaneuvering them.

Fifteen balls are racked in a triangle. The numbers have no meaning. Before the break each player chooses one of the two corner pockets at the foot of the table. Whoever makes eight balls in his pocket first, wins. If you make a ball in your opponent's pocket, it counts for him. If you make a ball in your pocket and a ball in his on the same shot, you both get credit for a ball and you keep shooting. If you make a ball in your pocket and on the same stroke a ball drops in one of the four unassigned pockets, it is spotted when you miss . . . unless it is the winning ball, in which case it is spotted when the table is clear to give you a chance to complete your run and win the game.

Tight defense is essential. Players try to "herd" balls toward their pockets without leaving each other a shot. It is frequently wiser to pass up a chance to score in favor of knocking balls away from your opponent's pocket. If your opponent leaves a ball so deep in the jaws of his pocket that it can't be knocked away, it might be best to make it yourself to deny him the opportunity of using it to get position on other balls, or to make it and scratch so that it is spotted instead of credited to him.

The game is so rich in both strategy and tactics that a book could be written about it. This is not that book. Try *Upscale One-Pocket,* by Jack Koehler (Sportology Publications, 1995).

Rotation

Rack the balls in a triangle with the 1 at the apex and the 2 and 3 at the other corners. The breaker must hit the 1-ball first to score . . . if he misses it, any pocketed balls are spotted behind the foot spot and the second player shoots from the resulting position. On every shot the shooter must hit the lowest-numbered ball

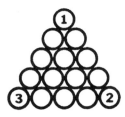

on the table . . . if he does and a ball goes in, any ball, he scores the value of the ball. Because the numbers on the fifteen balls total 120, the winner is the first player to score 61.

If a player contacts the lowest-numbered ball, makes a ball, and causes other balls to jump off the table, it is not a foul. The jumped balls are spotted and the inning continues. Otherwise, any ball leaving the table ends the inning.

Eight-ball

Eight-ball is the most widely played pool game, though nine-ball is gaining. It is often the first and only pool game people learn, and is the usual choice for coin-op tables and tavern leagues. Tavern owners think the game is wonderful because sometimes only minutes elapse before more coins are required. The game is played under a wide variety of rules. Mine follow.

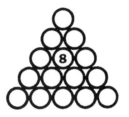

To win, you must pocket all the balls lower than 8, or all those higher than 8, followed by the 8. The players have a choice of either group of seven balls until a ball is made. If the first ball made is, for example, from the low group, the shooter is confined to the low balls for the rest of the game while his opponent is confined to the high balls. If the first ball that goes in is accompanied by a ball from the other group, the shooter retains his choice of groups and his inning continues. Slop counts except when shooting the 8, which must be called.

You lose if you make the 8 on the break and scratch, jump the 8 off the table at any time, scratch when shooting the 8, pocket the 8 when shooting at another ball, or make the 8 in a pocket other than the one you called. You win if you make the 8 on the break without scratching, which rarely happens because it is always racked in the middle of the fifteen balls.

It is a foul and your inning ends if you fail to drive a ball to a rail or fail to make the cueball hit a rail after hitting a ball. After a foul your opponent has the choice of taking the resulting position or having the cueball in hand. After a foul on the 8-ball there is the additional option of ball in hand with the 8-ball spotted.

An opponent's ball that goes in always stays down.

A little-known rule: If on the first scoring stroke a player makes one ball from one group and two from another, he has the two-ball group for the rest of the game.

A seldom-followed rule (even though it is in the Billiard Congress of America's rule book): Balls pocketed on the break do not determine the breaker's group; he shoots again and retains the choice.

Popular variations include banking the 8, making it in the same pocket as the last ball from the shooter's group, and restricting the 1-ball to one side pocket and the 15-ball to the other.

Remember, these are simply my unofficial rules; there are many others. For details on thirty-three pool and billiard games, consult the BCA rule book.

Bad hit—Hitting the wrong ball first.

Ball in hand—After a foul, the freedom to place the cueball anywhere behind the head string or, in many games, the freedom to place it anywhere on the table.

Billiard—1. Sending the cueball off one ball into another. 2. A one-point score in billiards (as opposed to pool).

Bridge—1. The hand on the table supporting the cue shaft. 2. The distance between the bridge and the tip of the cue.

Call shot—A style of play in which a ball and pocket are designated before shooting.

Carom—Deflecting one ball off another.

Combination—A shot in which the cueball drives one ball into another.

Diamonds—Small white disks set into the rails of most pool and billiard tables.

English—Cueball spin other than natural forward roll, such as sidespin, topspin, or backspin.

Foot rail—The rail at the end of the table where the balls are racked.

Foot spot—Point marked on the cloth two diamonds from the center of the foot rail.

Foul—An infraction of the rules that ends a player's inning.

Freeze, froze, frozen—Terms used to describe balls that are touching.

Grip—The part of the cue butt held by the "grip" hand.

Head rail—The end of the table where a player stands to start a game.

Head string—Imaginary line crossing the table two diamonds from the head rail.

Hooked—When the cueball's path to a designated ball is blocked.

Inning—A turn at the table.

Lagging for break—A method of determining who takes the first shot of a game. Each player places a ball behind the head string and banks it off the foot rail. The player whose ball stops closest to the head rail wins.

Massé shot—Striking the cueball off center with a steeply elevated cue to distort the cueball's path.

Scratch—In pool, accidentally sending the cueball into a pocket. In billiards, accidentally scoring a point.

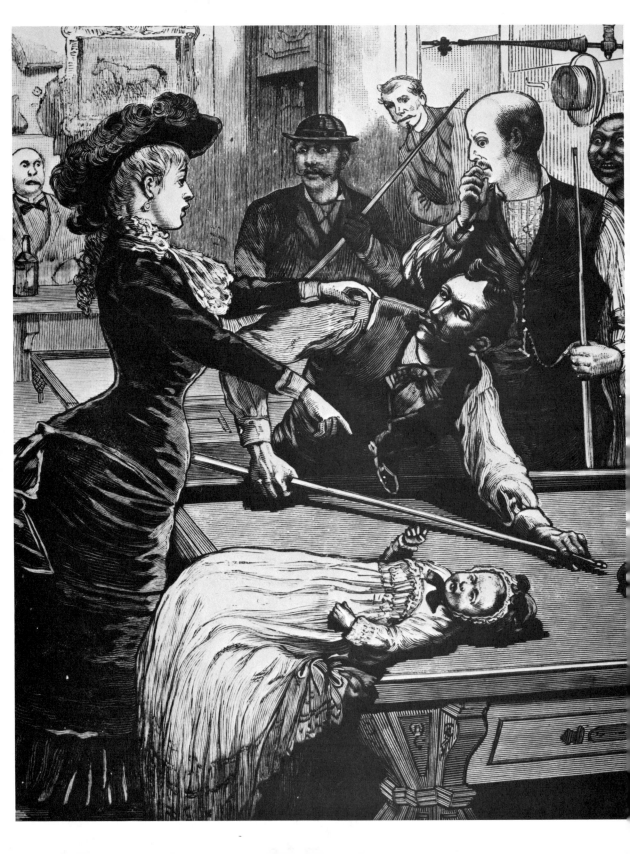

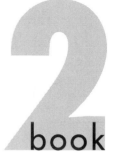
book

THREE-CUSHION BILLIARDS

To her dissolute husband, she cried: "You've played for everything else, now play for the baby."
(*Illustrated Police News*, 1882)

introduction

Having extolled pool in Book One, I am now going to try to convert everyone to the beautiful, subtle, spectacular, challenging, exhilarating, exasperating, cruel, rewarding, elegant, and endlessly intriguing game of three-cushion billiards, which is played on a table without pockets. There is a lot to like about it. You don't have to stop every few minutes to rack balls. You don't have to worry about the other player running the game out without giving you a chance to shoot. Unlike pool and snooker, you can play three-cushion billiards all over Scandinavia, the low countries, western, eastern, and southern Europe, North Africa, South and Central America, Japan, and Indonesia. In some cities in the United States, it's hard to find a "billiard" room that has billiard (pocketless) tables.

The game requires of its practitioners a significant amount of creative ability, for the shots have to be imagined before they can be made. In every game, positions arise that have never been seen before by man or beast. It is a game of both delicacy and power; on some shots the cueball must travel only a few inches, on others more than forty feet. Like chess it is a game of infinite richness, with each move combining offense and defense. It takes years to learn to play expertly, but, also like chess, it can be enjoyed at any level.

When you make a point in three-cushion billiards, you know you've done something. Five points in a row fills a beginner with pride. National-class players feel good for a week if they manage a run of ten. Hardly more than a half-dozen men in the long history of human striving have run more than twenty.

Propelled by an expert, a billiard ball teaches physics and geometry as it traces patterns on the table, speeding up, slowing down, and changing directions in surprising ways; it takes on uncanny properties, not the least of which is an apparent knowledge of what it is supposed to do and where it is supposed to go. There is a quality of suspended animation about the game that I find most absorbing. Most pool shots are made or missed within the blink of an eye, while in billiards the outcome is often in doubt for as long as seven or eight seconds.

In pool, pinpoint accuracy is often required in hitting the object ball. In billiards it is more a matter of blending the hit with the other variables of speed, stroke, and spin, and there is plenty of disagreement on some shots on what blend is best. The mix of variables, even what shot to try when a choice is presented, is more often a matter of the player's personality than his knowledge of the game or his powers of analysis. Is he reckless or chicken, a craftsman or a show-off? Whole schools of thought have arisen on how the game should be played. Americans are noted for stressing defense, Latin Americans offense. The Japanese are trying to reduce guesswork by refining the so-called diamond systems, while the Europeans are strong on position play.

There is disagreement on details, yes, but there is a large body of tested wisdom the student can acquire. Until the first publication of this book, however, hard and lengthy digging was required. A few things were revealed by Willie Hoppe in his 1941 *Billiards As It Should Be Played,* but the bulk of the iceberg remained submerged in a pool of oral lore guarded by initiates. Hoppe's book contains only fifty tiny diagrams on three-cushion, half of which are devoted to an out-of-focus discussion of the diamond system, which he didn't use in his own play.

Considering that the game is more than a century old (billiards in general goes back perhaps five hundred years, but the first three-cushion tournament was held in St. Louis in 1878) and that it is a popular pastime in much of the civilized world, it is surprising how little was published on technique. There was a near conspiracy of silence among some of the early great players, who carried secrets with them to the grave. Even today, little is available on such vital topics as safeties, kisses, position play, and how the diamond system really works. Scores of shots and stratagems have never before been diagrammed, written about, or even named in any language.

My aim in preparing a comprehensive guide to three-cushion billiards is to take the mystery out of it, to show that it is not as hopelessly abstract as outsiders sometimes think, to provide a system of nomenclature, to improve the play of those who already know the game and would like to know it better, and to make its pleasures available to pool players who don't have an expert handy whose brains they can pick (or who have one handy they can't stand). What follows is designed to shorten and simplify the process of teaching as well as learning the game. Readers who want to see the diagrammed shots demonstrated or who want to see the game played at the top level should contact a friendly local tournament player. For the name of the one nearest you, call the pool emporiums in your area and ask if they have billiard tables (some desk people don't know the difference between pool and billiard tables), or write to the United States Billiard Association, whose address is in the appendix. A good teacher, one who "sees" the shots and knows how to play them, is essential in learning a game that involves so many layers. Once you get the hang of it, though, it's easier than it looks. Some of the shots diagrammed here have to be seen to be believed.

In 1992 Accu-Stats Video Productions (see the appendix for address) began videotaping the annual international three-cushion tournaments hosted by 1993 world champion Sang Chun Lee at his S. L. Billiards in New York. Since then, Accu-Stats has built up a remarkable library of matches between the world's greatest players, taped close-up with commentary by (ahem!) yours truly. The tapes are a tremendous resource for learning the game that was unavailable to earlier generations of students. Even nonplayers, not to mention pool players, become mesmerized watching the great artists like Torbjorn Blomdahl of Sweden, the legendary Raymond Ceulemans of Belgium, Dick Jaspers of The Netherlands, Semih Sayginer of Turkey, and our own Sang Lee.

The beauty and elegance of one of the world's most visual and dramatic games has so far gone undetected by American television producers. However, beach volleyball, synchronized swimming, Wrestlemania, rhythmic gymnastics, bowling, and even fishing will be covered as usual.

Three-cushion rules

Three-cushion billiards is played on a pocketless table with two white balls and a red ball. One of the white balls, marked by a dot and called the black ball, is used by one player throughout the game as his cueball; the other player uses the other white ball as his cueball. A white-yellow-and-red ball combination is also popular.

To score a point, the cueball must hit three or more cushions and one of the object balls, in any sequence, before it hits the other object ball. Phrased another way: The cueball must hit both object balls, but before it gets to the second one it must hit three or more cushions. It is not necessary to hit three *different* cushions.

The first player to make an agreed-upon number of points wins. Friendly games are usually set at twenty-five, tournament games continue to thirty-five, forty, fifty, or sixty.

The international rules that now prevail around the world differ slightly from those Americans learned as children. Under international rules, when the cueball is frozen to a ball only the two balls are respotted . . . unless the player chooses to shoot away from the frozen ball. When respotting, the shooter's cueball goes on the head spot, the opponent's cueball goes on the center spot, and the red ball goes on the foot spot. If the third ball (the one not frozen to the cueball) interferes with the spotting of one of the frozen balls, the ball being spotted goes on the spot assigned to the interfering ball. Under old American rules, the player confronted with a frozen cueball has the option of taking the opening break shot.

The position for the opening break shot is given in Diagram 142.

Deliberate safeties are banned under the new rules—you must always take a shot that has at least *some* chance of scoring, and points are not deducted from anybody's score for any reason. Old American rules permitted one deliberate safety, after which the player had to make an effort to score or risk losing a point. Under international rules, a foul ends the shooter's inning, and he loses nothing but his aplomb. Old rules OK'd knocking an object ball off the table—it was respotted and the inning continued if a point was scored. Now the inning ends when any ball leaves the table.

Be sure to find out what local practice is before engaging in a contest for a significant wager.

preliminaries

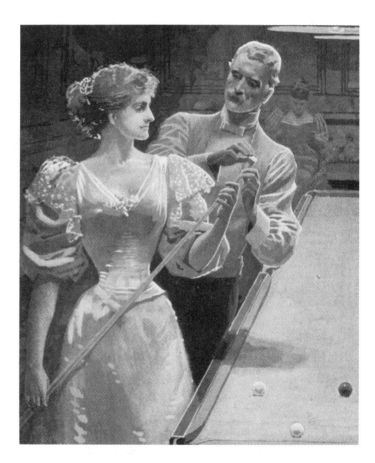

From *Billiards*, by Major W. Broadfoot, R.E.
Longmans, Green and Co., London and Bombay, 1896
Illustrated by Lucien Davies, R.I.

If it weren't for the substantial margin of error on many shots, three-cushion billiards would be too taxing to be enjoyable. As it is, the target the cueball must find to score is often several times wider than the width of the second object ball, which makes the game a little easier than it might seem to a passerby.

A second object ball in the middle of the table presents a target twice as wide as its own width because the cueball can hit thin on either side. Move it to within a few inches of a rail and its size as a target is much increased because the cueball can either hit it directly or bounce into it off the rail, provided that the cueball has struck the other ball and three or more rails before approaching. Positioned in a corner about three inches from each rail, a ball as a final target is a foot wide.

A ball near a rail or in a corner is called a big ball, and finding ways to take advantage of it is the most overriding consideration in selecting a shot.

In this section the "big-ball principle" will be explained in some detail and the reader will be given initial exposure to a few standard three-cushion shot patterns, concepts, and terms.

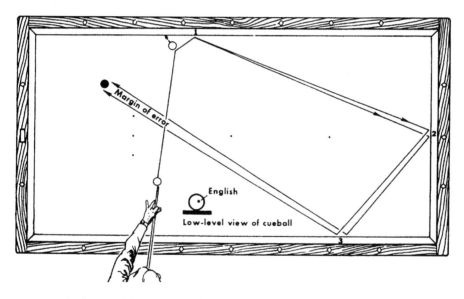

1 Around-the-table natural

This is a very common three-cushion shot pattern. It's called a natural because running English is used without a hard stroke and because the rails are struck in adjacent order. Because the second object ball is not near a rail, it is, as a target, twice as wide as its diameter, or 4⅞ inches.

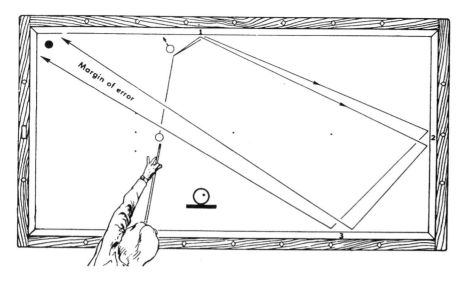

2 The biggest possible ball

See how much greater is the margin of error when the second ball is in a corner (but not frozen to both rails, which would make it smaller as a target than the ball in the previous diagram). Note that the rails are numbered in the order contacted. Note also that the lines represent the paths taken by the center of the balls, which is why they do not touch the rails or other balls. This method of diagramming, never used before the first edition of this book was published in 1978, permits the depiction of true lines of aim and travel. (Lines connecting contact points are very misleading.)

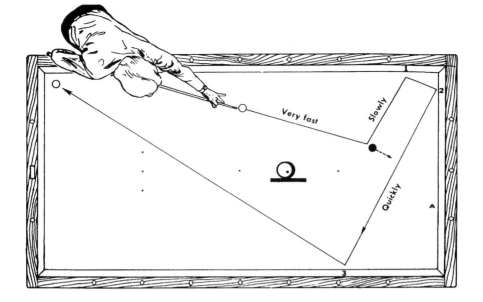

3 Spin shot to a big ball

This shot could be made by hitting the red thin on the right side (as the shooter faces the ball), contacting the first rail at point A, the second rail near the number 3, and the third rail near the white ball. (The ball that is not the red ball and not the cueball will be called the white ball, or the white.) Because the white is a big ball, however, the better way is to shoot a spin shot, about which more later. Hit the red ball full with low right, drawing the cueball to the side rail. The spin adds speed to the cueball as it caroms out of the corner.

In this diagram the enlarged inset of the cueball shows both the exact English to use and the amount of red ball to hit. In most of the diagrams in Book Two, the amount of ball to hit will be indicated only by the dashed arrow showing the direction the object ball takes. The dashed arrow is meant to show direction only, not distance. Tracing the entire path of the first object ball with a dashed line would clutter the diagrams too much.

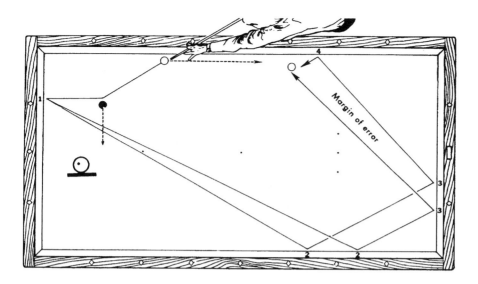

4 End rail to a big ball

There are two ways to play this shot. Beginners are apt to shoot the cueball along the dashed line, trying to score with the pattern given in Diagram 1. But the white ball is a big ball if a way can be found to hit the red and three rails before approaching it. Such a way is given. Note the comfortable margin of error.

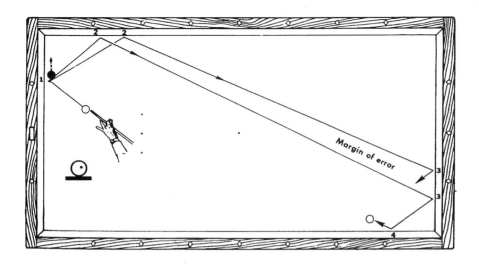

5 Another end rail to a big ball

If the "hole" between the white ball and the rail is small—say, less than three inches—a good policy is to aim for it because it represents the center of the target. If the hole is large enough to let the cueball pass through easily without scoring the point, then you must choose one of the two scoring paths and try to follow it.

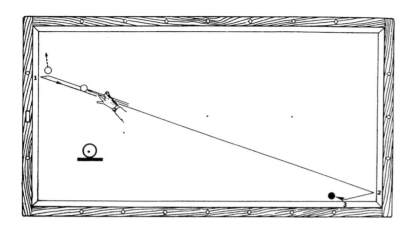

6 Drop-in back-up

Not enough right English can be applied here to make the cueball follow the scoring path given in the previous diagram, so something else must be tried. The shot diagrammed is quite difficult because the target on the third rail is very narrow. This is an example of a "small ball." The shot must be hit softly to make sure the cueball doesn't back up steeply off the second rail directly into the red, missing the third rail.

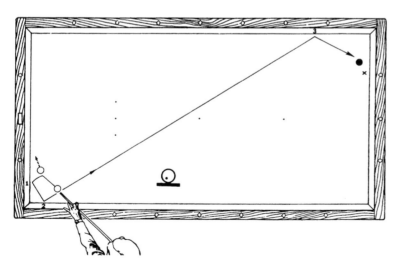

7 Diagonal draw to a big ball

Don't try to hit point X for the third rail. Use more draw and follow the path diagrammed, which makes the red a big ball.

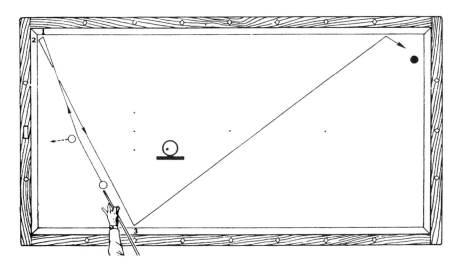

8 Fan the ball around the table

Here the attempt to adopt the previous pattern is too difficult, but there is another way to make the red ball "big." Hit the object ball extremely thin as shown with extreme left English. Not much force is required because the cueball transfers hardly any speed to the first ball.

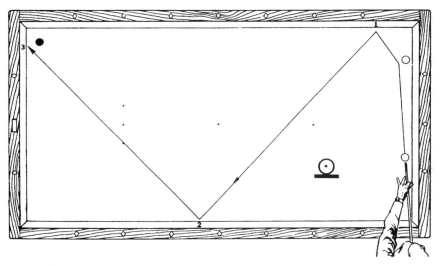

9 Outside zigzag

The red is a big ball but there is no way to use it as such. The best shot is the one diagrammed. Because this rail can also be picked up on the other side of the red, this can be called a "two-way" shot.

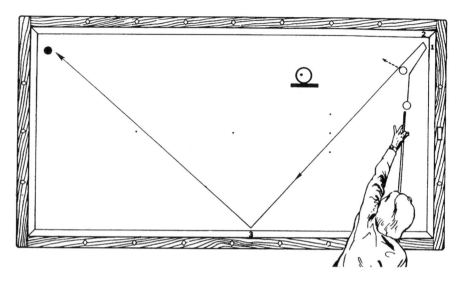

10 Inside zigzag

Much easier than the previous shot because an extra rail can be hit at the outset allowing the cueball to score on a wide target. The angle off the third rail is hard to judge because hold-up is not as predictable as running English. This pattern is well worth practicing.

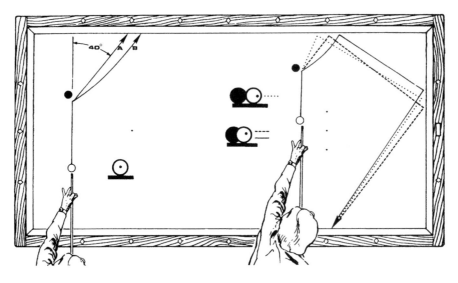

11 The half-ball hit

If the cueball is aimed directly at the edge of an object ball and is stroked rather softly without follow or draw, the path is deflected by 34 degrees, as shown by line A. A harder stroke sends the cueball along B. The half-ball hit is important because the amount of deflection is less sensitive to error than other hits—that is, hitting the object ball slightly fuller or slightly thinner will still result in a deflection of close to 34 degrees. The player who can accurately estimate the half-ball angle can eliminate one variable on many shots, leaving only speed and English to be considered. For more, see pages 45–47 in *Byrne's Advanced Technique.*

Blending variables

The right side of the diagram is intended to show that the same point can be reached on the third rail by a variety of paths. The dotted line is for a thin hit, slow speed, and extreme right English. The dashed line is for a half-ball hit and running English. The solid line results from a fuller hit and more speed and follow.

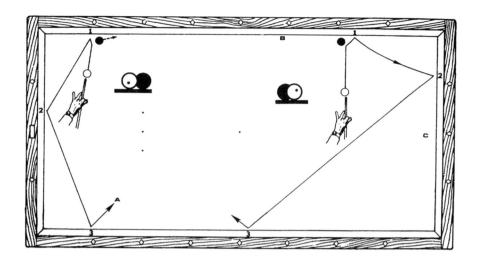

12 Draw off a rail

When the first ball is close to a rail, hitting the cueball below center holds it on a straight path, as seen at the left. A point would be scored if the second ball were at A, B, or, with enough speed, C.

Follow off a rail

At the right is the effect of follow off a ball on the rail. With this action, characterized by a curved path between the first and second rails, it is possible to send the cueball far up the third rail.

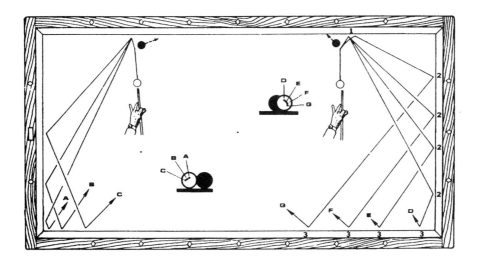

13 Varying English only

At the left the red ball is cut thin. The more English is used, the more the cue-ball jumps to the left off the first rail. At the right is a half-ball hit. The exact paths given here are not meant to be memorized, only the principle.

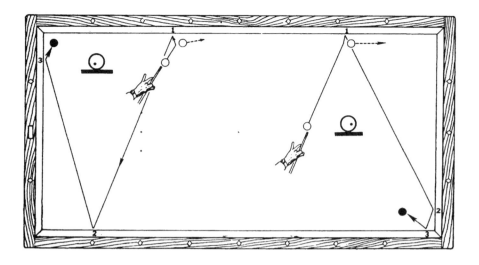

14 Natural and reverse shots

The shot at the right is called a short angle—short angle because it takes place on one end of the table only (the so-called "short" table, two diamonds wide and four diamonds long)—and natural because the cueball has running English as it hits three adjacent rails.

The shot at the left is not called a natural because the cueball has hold-up English on the second and third rails. Neither shot is considered difficult. The patterns recur so frequently that the student must learn to judge them accurately.

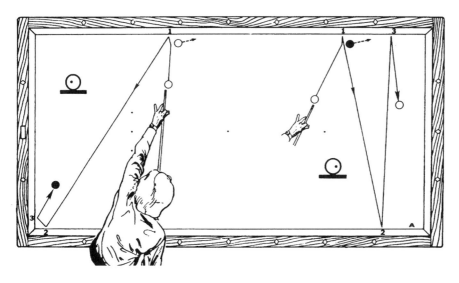

15 Short-angle back-up

The term back-up is used for the shot at the left because the cueball "backs up" out of the corner with hold-up English.

Twice across

The twice-across or cross-table shot is shown at the right. A slightly elevated cue keeps the cueball moving down the table in a zigzag pattern. The shot could also be made as a back-up by using more English and sending the cueball into the second rail at A, then off the end rail to the white.

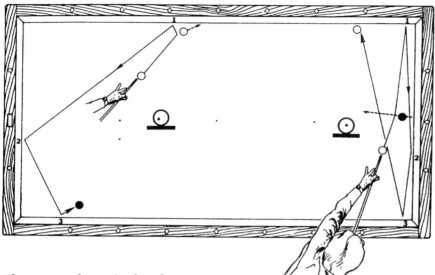

16 Short-angle spin-back

The shot at the left requires left English and a full hit. Hitting a ball full with English removes much of the cueball's speed but little of its English. The cueball in this case arrives at the second rail with a lot of spin in relation to its forward speed, which is why it must be directed at a point on the second rail farther from the corner than neophytes suppose.

The flat short angle

Not all shots require English. The one at the right is played with a centerball hit. Even a trace of right English will throw the cueball too far to the right off the first rail. In aiming such a shot, special attention must be given to the exact point the tip will contact the cueball.

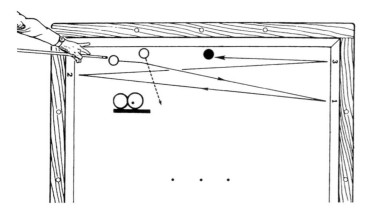

17 "Manufactured angle" twice across

When there is no natural angle for a shot, an angle can sometimes be "manufac-tured" with draw, follow, or English. This cross-table pattern is familiar to every good player. The "backward" angle off the first rail is best achieved with low left English. If the cueball comes off the first rail properly, it follows a path similar to that at the right of Diagram 15. Some speed is needed on this one.

twenty ball-first patterns 2

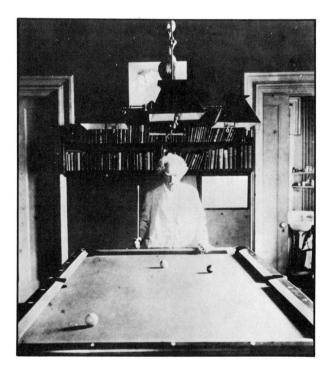

Mark Twain.
(The Mark Twain Memorial)

A large majority of shots that come up in a typical game of three-cushion are played by hitting a ball first rather than one or more rails. In this section twenty-one of the most commonly encountered ball-first patterns are diagrammed and discussed. The exact position of the balls is not important. What the student must learn to recognize are the *patterns,* because the balls never come to rest in exactly the same position twice.

Not all of the shots shown are easy to make, but that's no reason to become discouraged. The best players in the country miss on half of their attempts.

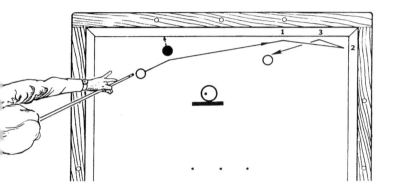

18 Cut shot double-the-rail

Shoot softly for maximum effect.

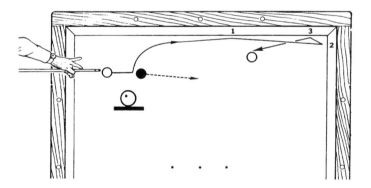

19 Force-follow double-the-rail

This takes a good stroke, but the action is beautiful to see when it works. Don't shoot so hard that the cueball hits the first rail before bending forward.

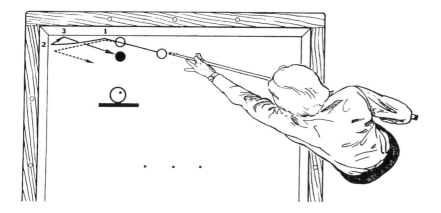

20 Smash-through double-the-rail

Much easier than the previous shot, partly because it doesn't have to be hit so hard. Some abject beginners can make this with the right coaching. On shots requiring more than a little English, make sure your tip is properly groomed and chalked.

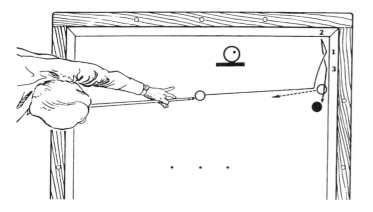

21 Snake shot

So-called because of the writhing action. Hit the white as full as you can without getting a double-kiss. Often missed through the use of too much speed. Don't spare the English and follow on this and the previous two shots.

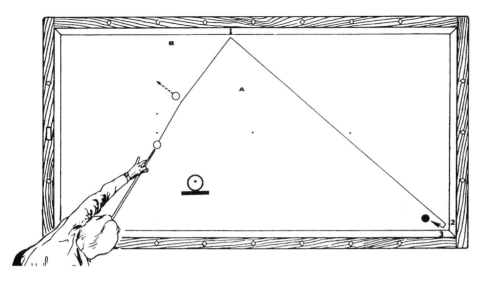

22 Fan the ball into the corner

When I say fan the ball, I mean hit it really thin. On some shots of this type the cueball goes twenty feet and the first object ball three inches. Note that the same pattern could be used if the second ball were at A or B. Since an objective here is to come off the first rail rather sharply, don't use running English. Don't use hold-up English, either, except in an emergency, because it is always difficult to judge.

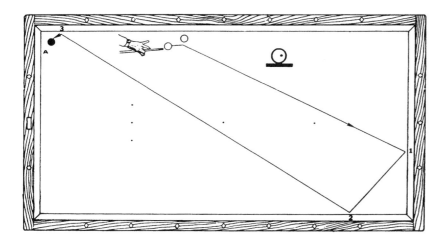

23 Outside cut around the table

The red ball is big but there is no way to make use of it, except by a chancy force follow straight into the white. In the diagram, the cueball is sent "outside" the first ball, that is, on the side toward the center of the table. Decide in advance whether to play the shot as drawn or into point A for the third rail. The decision depends on kisses, position, and safety, which will be taken up later. The shot can also be played as a draw-back cross-table (Diagram 14, left).

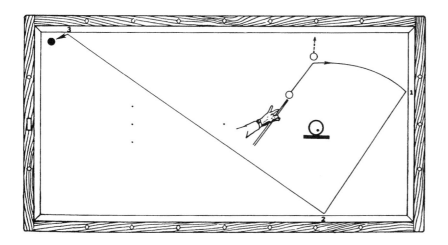

24 Outside draw around the table

A variation of the previous pattern. The cueball path must be bent by draw off the first ball to establish the correct angle of approach to the first rail.

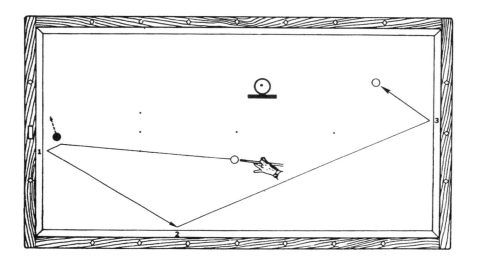

25 Long angle

Good players differ slightly in the blend of hit, speed, and spin they use on this shot. When the cueball is this far from the first ball, it is best to use little or no English to eliminate the need for estimating curve.

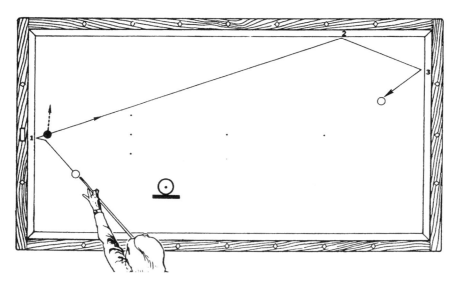

26 Long angle drop-in

The shooter has a choice of this pattern or the previous one. The pattern here is preferred because it is easier to estimate where the second rail must be hit.

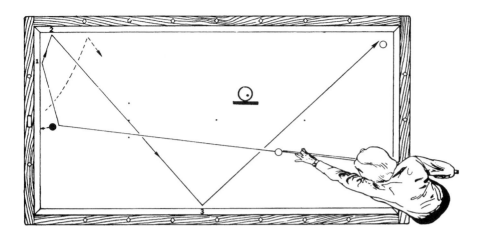

27 Off-the-end zigzag

Not too tough if the white is big in the corner. When the first ball is more than the width of a ball or two from the end rail, draw is needed to send the cueball into the first rail close to the corner. When the first ball is closer than that, use follow to bend the cueball path between the first and second rail as shown by the dashed line (an application of the action portrayed in Diagram 12, right).

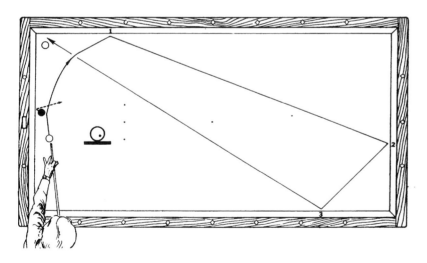

28 Manufactured angle around the table

Here draw is used to establish the proper angle into the first rail. The thin hit on the red ball is needed to avoid an immediate kiss. (If the red ball was frozen to the rail, a deliberate kiss could be made use of. See the examples in Diagrams 120–123.)

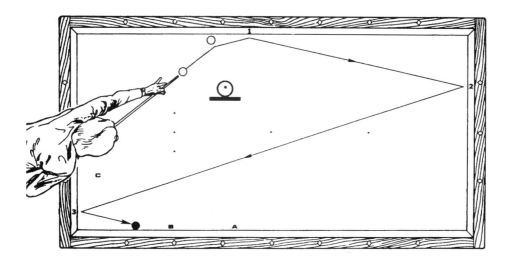

29 Side rail up-and-down

Because the red is frozen to the rail, the third-rail target is too small for a short-angle spin-back (Diagram 16). It can be tried, but better is the no-English or high-English up-and-down diagrammed here. The red can be at B or A or even farther up the side rail.

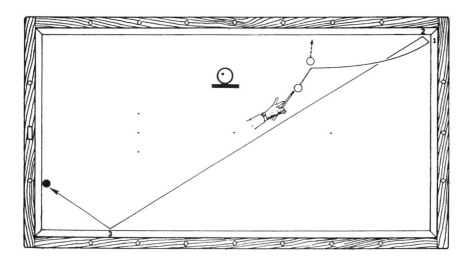

30 The corner plunge

The amount of curve into the first rail can be adjusted by varying the hit, speed, and follow.

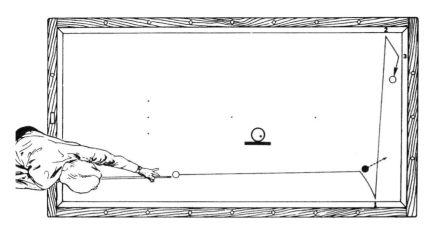

31 Reverse cross-table

Beginners rarely see this shot and usually can't handle it when they do, which isn't surprising because it's a severe test even for good players. When planning the shot, pick a reasonable contact point on the first rail, then apply enough spin to the cueball to make it follow the required path from there to the second rail. The cueball must still be spinning when it hits the second rail.

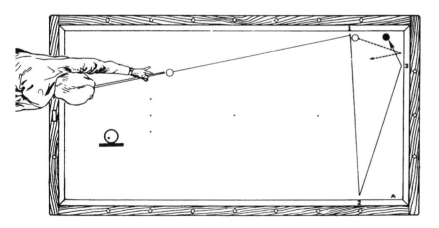

32 Twice-across reverse

The white ball can be as close as a quarter-inch from the rail—all you need is enough room to miss the kiss as shown. The shot is diagrammed with reverse English, which is why the cueball goes almost straight across the table, then spins off the second rail. It can also be made with a thinner hit and plain draw, sending the cueball to the second rail at A.

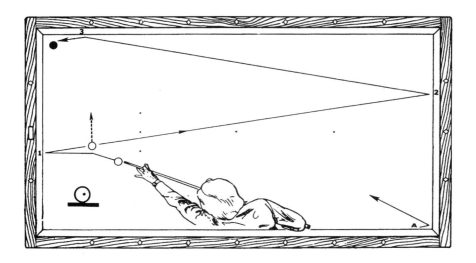

33 End rail up-and-down

There are three choices here: twice across off the right side of the white in the style of Diagram 15, right; up and down as diagrammed; or the long angle to the side rail at A. The long angle is impossible with natural English when the contact point on the end rail is to the right of the nameplate.

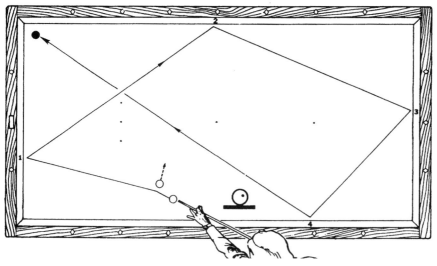

34 Running four-railer

Not difficult if the red is big in the corner. With a thin hit there should be no kiss.

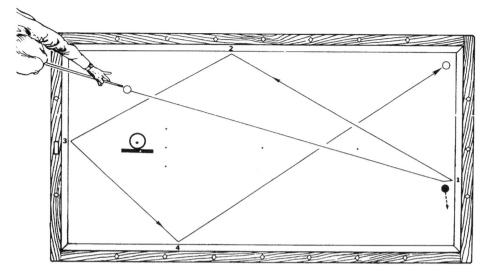

35 Ball-on-rail four-railer

A common pattern and not easy when the cueball is so far from the first ball. Hit the cueball slightly below center and slightly left. Less ball and more English is possible but it creates the problem of allowing for curve.

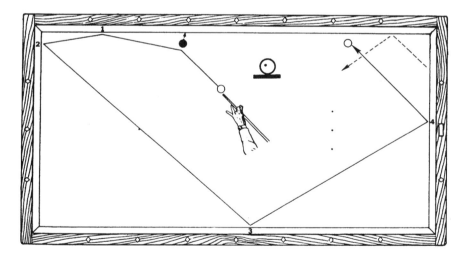

36 Long around-the-table natural

With running English on shots of this type it is hard to get beyond the second diamond from the corner on the fifth rail. All you have to do is make sure you don't miss the shot "short," that is, along the dashed line. There is a kiss to beat just to the left of the shooter's elbow.

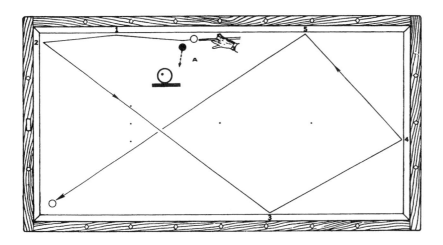

37 Inside five-railer

The cueball has to travel a long way here, but that's not hard if you can hit the first ball thin. The same pattern off the other side of the red, from cueball position A, I call an outside five-railer. In many cases it's easier to score by going five or even seven rails instead of three.

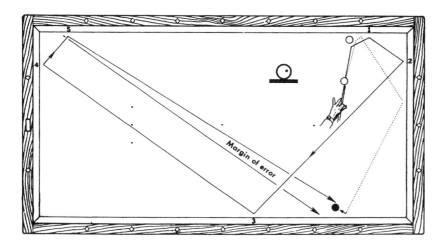

38 Short angle versus twice-around

The player can go three rails along the dotted line or five rails along the solid line. If the red is more than two ball-widths from the rail, the short angle is best, but positioned as it is, the red is a big ball on the five-rail pattern. To be weighed in the choice are chances of position and a kiss-out.

3

seventeen rail-first patterns

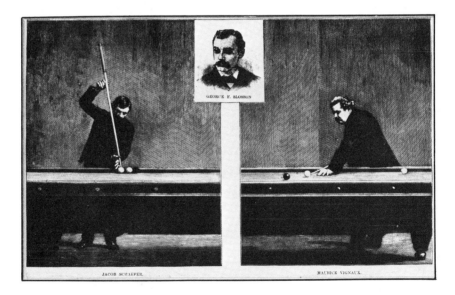

Harper's Weekly, 1885.
(Byrne Collection)

When one ball is near a rail or a corner, it is often far easier to score by hitting one or two rails first, and when all three balls are near the same rail, there is often a double-the-rail, three-cushion-first possibility. This section covers seventeen of the most common rail-first patterns. Not included are natural three-cushion banks, which will be discussed in the following section on diamond systems.

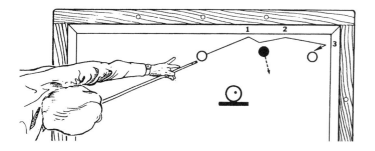

39 Ticky

One of the easiest shots in billiards. Use running English, hit the rail before the ball, and shoot softly. It's not so easy when the distance between the first ball and the rail is much less than a ball-width or more than three or four ball-widths. The student, through practice, must become friendly with this pattern because varieties of it come up over and over again.

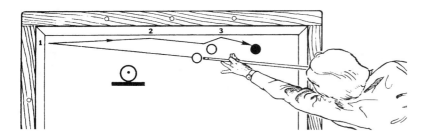

40 Back-up ticky

No English is required or desired for this two-rail-first shot when the balls are placed as shown.

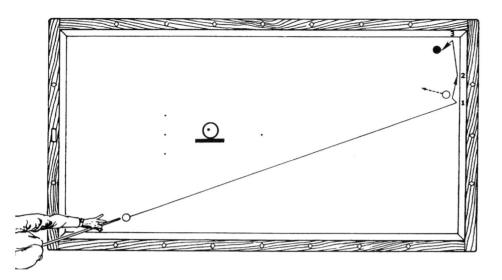

41 Long-range ticky

It would be a crime to overlook an easy shot like this in view of the difficulty of all the other options.

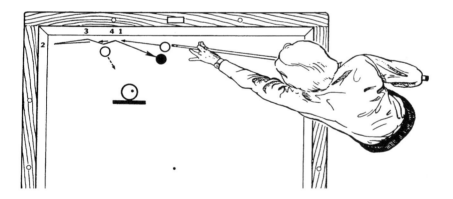

42 Double-the-rail back-up ticky

Shoot through the hole with double-the-rail English and make a back-up ticky like the one in Diagram 40.

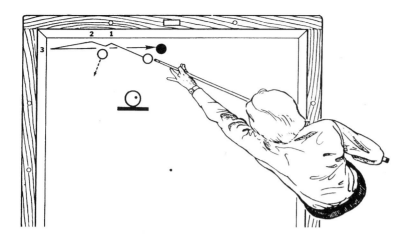

43 Hold-up ticky

A valuable shot. The hold-up English brings the cueball off the third rail at an unnatural angle. In this pattern the cueball hits every cushion with hold-up English.

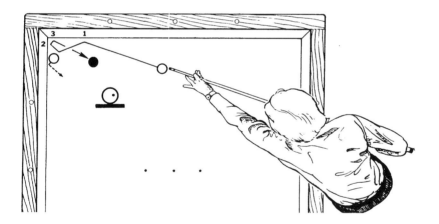

44 Corner spin-out

Easy when you get the hang of it. Here the English is hold-up on the first rail, running on the next two.

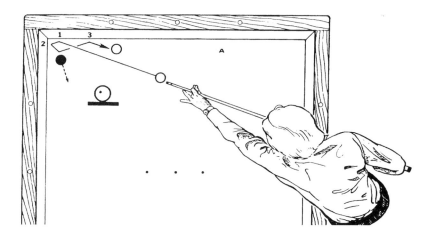

45 Corner snap-back

The previous pattern can be used here, but when the first ball is off the rail, it is often better to use what Col. E. J. "Stub" Pilotte of the United States Air Force calls snap-back action. If the second ball is at A, use less running English and try for a little less of the first ball.

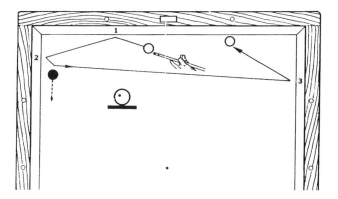

46 Corner cross-table

Similar to the last pattern, but there the English was hold-up off the third rail; here it is running all the way. Sometimes you'll catch another rail just before the second ball.

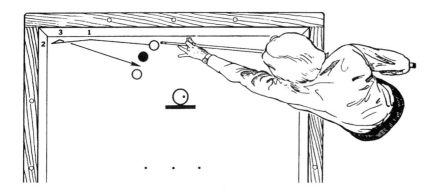

47 Double-the-rail

Sometimes this is duck soup, a characterization I may regret if this book is translated into Japanese. Usually best to hit the first rail close to the corner to minimize the amount of English needed.

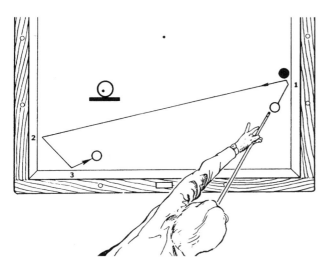

48 Rail-first draw-back cross-table

The less red is hit, the more draw is required to bring the cueball back at the required angle. A full hit is best, even though more force is needed initially, because the cueball will enter the left corner with a high ratio of spin to speed, which enlarges the area on the third rail that the cueball can hit and still make the point.

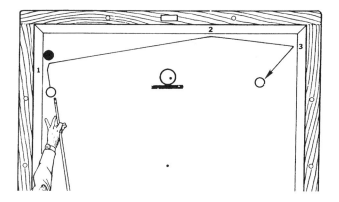

49 Rail-first short angle

A relatively easy shot that should be mastered. If the cueball is a foot to the right, no draw is needed.

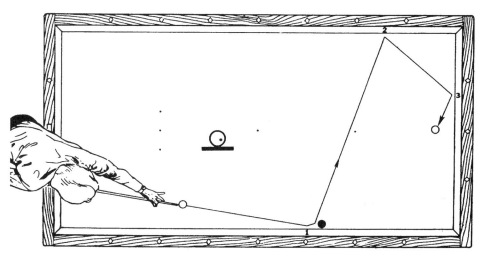

50 Rail-first reverse cross-table

The pattern here is not particularly mysterious—the running spin off the second rail is the main feature—but accuracy is hard to achieve. Speed makes a big difference because the faster the cueball arrives at the first rail, the more it compresses the rubber, which changes the angle at which the cueball hits the red. At the start of my mildly distinguished career as a player, I asked the great Welker Cochran how to calculate the hit on this shot and also the one in Diagram 186. "Shoot them a hundred times," the master said, "and then you'll know."

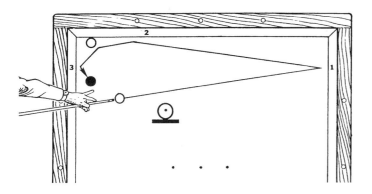

51 Two-rail cross-table bank

A fairly high-percentage shot when the balls are arranged like this. No English is needed, so make sure none is applied.

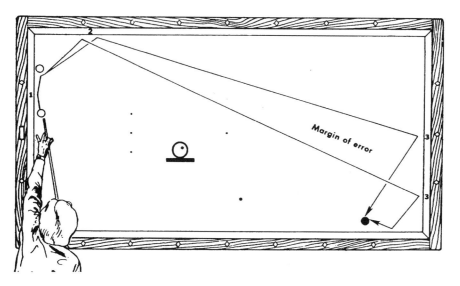

Margin of error

52 End rail first to a big ball

Someone who is just beginning or who is not terribly bright might go off the right side of the white and hope for a third rail just before hitting the red. Rail first is much better because the red then becomes a big ball. For the largest possible margin of error, come off the rail and hit the white full instead of thin so that the cue-ball travels up the table with a high spin-to-speed ratio. That way the target on the third rail that can be hit is at least a foot wide.

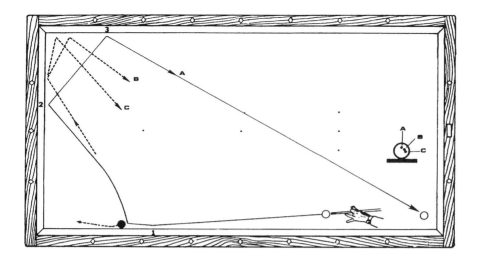

53 Side rail first to a big ball

Study this diagram well. It shows clearly how English affects a rail-first shot. With the same hit off the rail on the red ball, the cueball will trace the A, B, or C paths, depending on the English. Follow makes the path bend forward between the first and second rail and is the best way to reach a ball in the corner, as diagrammed.

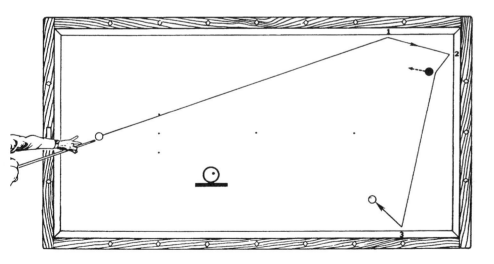

54 Inside umbrella

For seventy years at least this shot has been called, for some reason, the umbrella. It's tough, but it has to be resorted to on occasion. Some players like it and are therefore good at it, or vice versa.

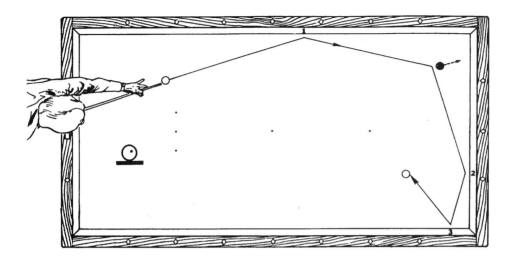

55 Outside umbrella

The angle off the first rail must be estimated with precision. To facilitate that, shoot softly.

diamond systems

4

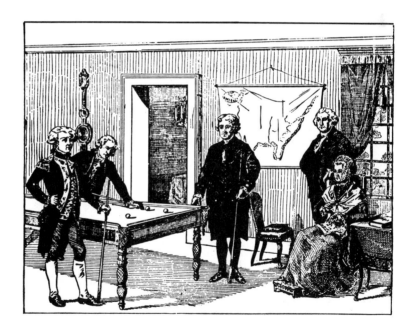

The Founding Fathers.
(*Modern Billiards*, 1881)

Counting diamonds and applying rules of geometry and arithmetic will not enable you to become a mechanical scoring machine. There are number systems that are helpful in aiming certain kinds of shots, particularly bank shots, but they must be modified at every turn by the fruits of experience. They require close control of speed and English, which is why they work best for players who are also good at other phases of the game. Many very fine players rely almost totally on judgment; others who use the system with great success make slight adjustments, sometimes unconsciously, I believe, when their instincts tell them that the formula isn't going to quite work.

When a ball is banked around a table, many factors influence the angles at which it caroms off the cushions, among them the initial speed, direction, and English, the height of the rails in relation to the diameter of the ball, the consistency, quality, and temperature of the rubber, the moisture content of the cloth, the type, condition, and nap of the cloth, and the trueness of the balls, cushions, and table. Yet the 1991 and earlier editions of the *Official Rules & Records Book* published by the Billiard Congress of America stated, laughingly I would hope, that the diamond system, as an "indisputable fact," "takes all the guesswork out of 3-cushion billiards." The *real* indisputable fact is that if you miss a system shot it isn't necessarily because you did something wrong or that I gave you the wrong information. Lots of valid excuses can be invoked.

Tables vary widely, not just one from another but sometimes from one rail to another. Tournament players faced with a strange table always devote part of their warm-up time to banking the cueball around in various directions—they are looking for inconsistencies, a short corner, for example—and they want to see how the angles compare with those on the equipment they are used to. They may have to make adjustments on many shots, especially system shots.

Having issued the above warnings and disclaimers, I will predict, nevertheless, that if you do not now use the system, and if you are not already an expert player, a close reading of this section will significantly improve your game, increasing your accuracy on many kinds of shots, not just bank shots.

There are many kinds of diamond systems. The one I will devote the most space to is called "the standard 5" or "the corner 5." It is applicable to a large family of shots, those in which the cueball is banked with running English off one side rail, an end rail, and the opposite side rail. To use it you have to be able to add and subtract in your head numbers less than eighty.

The system has been traditionally taught in the United States using fractions. Following the Japanese example, I use decimals because they are easier to manipulate. The Japanese call the first diamond 10 and the second 20, and so on. I feel it is more sensible to call the first diamond 1.0, so I have moved the decimal one place to the left.

Don't give up if you can't follow the explanation on first exposure. Stick to it. Some very dumb people have learned how to use the diamond system, which is hard to put in words.

The diamond system is based on a simple relationship between the contact point on the first rail, measured in diamonds from the far corner, the contact point on the third rail, measured the same way, and the effective point of origin of the cueball, measured as shown in Diagram 57. The second rail plays no part in the calculations.

Reference: More on diamond systems can be found in *Byrne's Advanced Technique* and *Byrne's Wonderful World* (Parts 3 and 6).

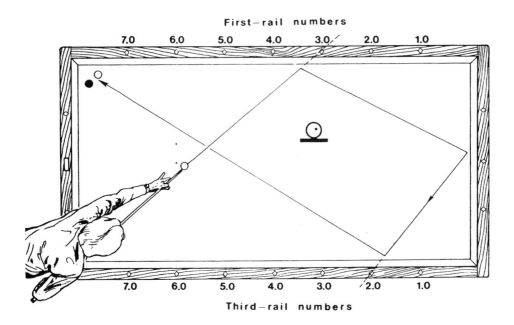

56 Numbering the first and third rails

When shooting around the table in this direction, the first and third rails are numbered in whole steps from the right end. If the cueball is shot with running English along a line that starts at the lower left corner and passes through diamond 3.0, then it will bounce off three rails and directly into the upper left corner. Note that the line of aim is directly at the inlaid spot on the wooden part of the rail, not at the point opposite it on the rubber. Note too that the path of the cueball, if extended after leaving the second rail, would pass through diamond 2.0 on the third rail. The projected paths are always extended through to the diamonds in the explanations that follow.

Try this pattern and adjust your speed and English until you can make the cueball hit within an inch or two of the corner.

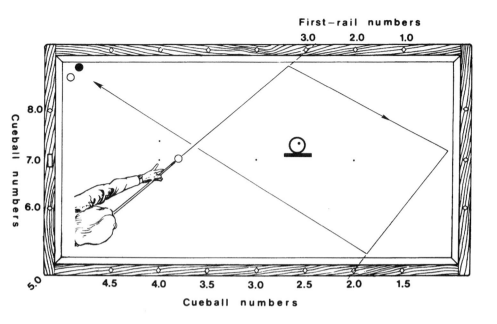

Cueball numbers

8.0

7.0

6.0

5.0   4.5   4.0   3.5   3.0   2.5   2.0   1.5

Cueball numbers

57 Numbering the cueball origin

Some forgotten hero seventy or eighty years ago had the idea of numbering the cueball origin points in such a way that a simple formula would be satisfied, namely, that the first-rail number, F, subtracted from the cueball number, C, equals the third-rail number, T, or $C-F=T$. Since shooting out of the corner to 3.0 leads to 2.0 on the third rail, the corner has to be given a value of 5.0 because 5.0 minus 3.0 equals 2.0.

It remained to assign numbers for all cueball origin points on the left short rail and the lower long rail. If you start the cueball on a line passing through the first diamond from the corner of the long rail, it turns out that you must shoot through to 2.5 on the first rail in order to hit 2.0 on the third; therefore, the cueball origin must be given the number 4.5. The first diamond from the corner on the short rail is called 6.0 because from there the cueball must be shot toward 4.0 on the first rail to reach 2.0 on the third. In this fashion a number can be found for every point of cueball origin. They are given in the above diagram. Note that along the short rail the numbers increase by 1.0 for each diamond and that along the long rail they decrease by 0.5.

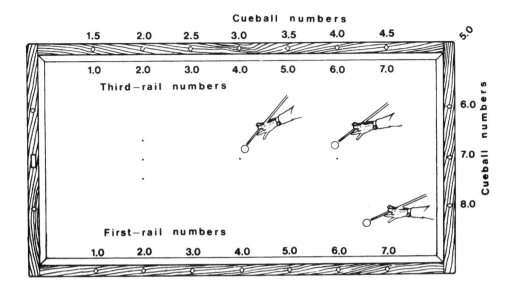

Cueball numbers

1.5   2.0   2.5   3.0   3.5   4.0   4.5   5.0

1.0   2.0   3.0   4.0   5.0   6.0   7.0

Third–rail numbers

6.0

7.0

Cueball numbers

8.0

First–rail numbers

1.0   2.0   3.0   4.0   5.0   6.0   7.0

58 Numbering from another corner

Any corner can be assigned the 5.0 cueball origin number depending on the direction of the bank. This diagram shows first-rail, third-rail, and cueball numbering for banks that begin in a generally southwesterly direction. Always start by deciding which is the basic cueball origin corner—call that corner 5.0 and continue the numbering from there. A possible source of confusion is that the third rail carries two sets of numbers. They must be kept separate in your mind.

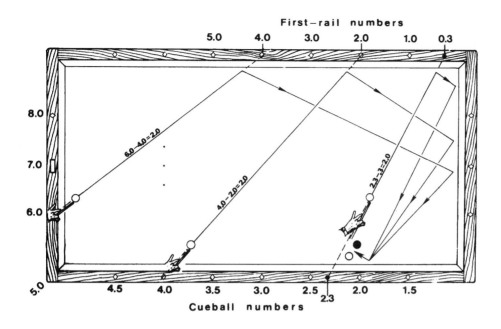

5.0   4.0   3.0   2.0   1.0   0.3

8.0

7.0

6.0

5.0

6.0-4.0=2.0

4.0-2.0=2.0

2.3-3=2.0

4.5   4.0   3.5   3.0   2.5   2.0   1.5
2.3

Cueball numbers

59 How to hit a third-rail point

The diagram shows how 2.0 on the third rail can be hit from three cueball positions. The cueball at the left is starting from 6.0. Since we know that T (third-rail number) equals 2.0 and C (cueball number) equals 6.0, F (first-rail number) must equal 4.0 because F = C – T.

The middle cueball is starting from 4.0. What number subtracted from 4.0 equals the desired destination, 2.0? The answer is 2.0, so shoot through to 2.0 on the first rail.

The line of aim for the cueball at the right is not so easy to find. You must try several lines of aim until you find one that satisfies the formula, estimating the values of points between the diamonds. In the example, 2.0 can be reached on the third rail by shooting from 2.3 to 0.3.

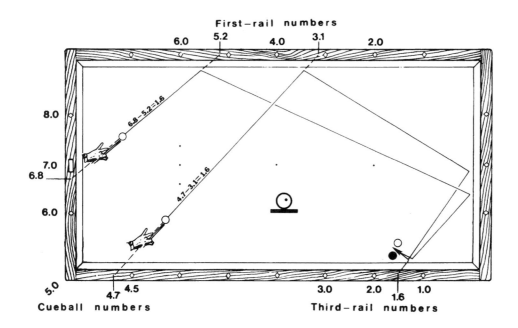

First-rail numbers

6.0   5.2   4.0   3.1   2.0

8.0

7.0
6.8

6.0

6.8 − 5.2 = 1.6

4.7 − 3.1 = 1.6

5.0   4.7   4.5   3.0   2.0   1.6   1.0

Cueball numbers   Third−rail numbers

60 How to hit another third-rail point

Let us assume that you have studied this position and have decided the point can be scored if the cueball leaves the second rail and heads for the imaginary point 1.6 on the third rail. Given are solutions for two cueball locations.

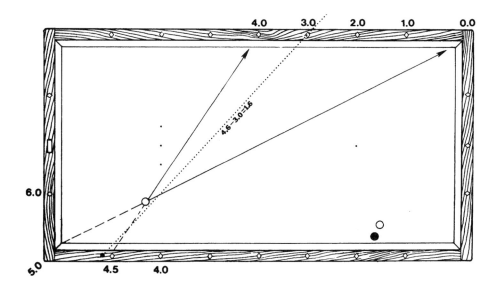

61 Finding the cueball position

It is important to understand that when the cueball is not on a rail its point of origin changes with the point of aim. Only when you aim the cueball somewhere can you determine the cueball number. Above is the same position as the second example in the previous diagram. Aiming the cueball at the corner (0.0), results in a cueball number of 5.0; aiming it at 4.0 gives 4.5.

In the example, the player is trying to find a cueball aiming line that will yield two numbers that differ by 1.6. One way to do it quickly is to lay your cue on the table along a path that satisfies the requirement and involves easy arithmetic. The dotted line is such a path. If you point the tip at 3.0 you immediately know that the butt should be laid across 4.6 to give a difference of 1.6. Pick up the cue, move it parallel to the path it was on until it is above the cueball, and you will find that you are on the 4.7–3.1 line, the line you seek.

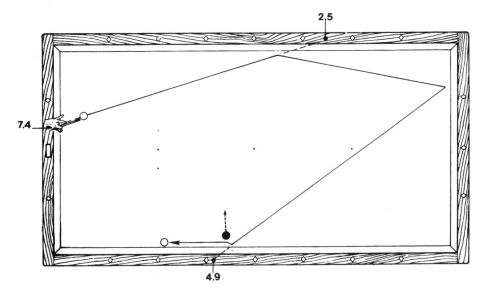

62 A long-angle bank

Shots of this type are often missed because the third-rail number isn't chosen properly. Even though the cueball will contact the rail about halfway between the 4.0 and 5.0 diamonds on the third rail, the third-rail number to use is 4.9 because the path must be extended until it intersects the imaginary spot on the wood between the diamonds.

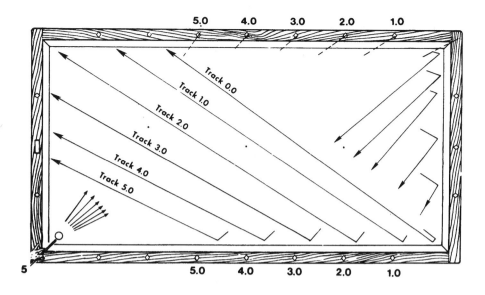

63 Third-rail returns, or tracks

When the object balls are close to the third rail, it is easy to select the proper third-rail target number. When they aren't, you must know what paths the cueball follows between the third and fourth rails. The paths are called third-rail returns, or tracks.

The tracks in this diagram for a cueball starting from the corner are basic and should be memorized. Your table, however, especially if it isn't covered with a high grade of imported cloth like Simonis from Belgium or Granito (made by Gorina) from Spain, may give different readings. Test your table and make a diagram like this for future reference.

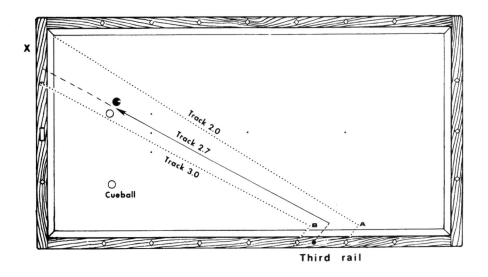

64 Locating the object balls

The first step in playing this shot three rails first with the aid of the diamond system is to find out what track the object balls are on. Stand at X and sight back to the third rail along the paths you have memorized in the previous diagram. Be sure to sight toward points A and B, which is where imaginary cueballs are when they carom off the third rail—don't sight through to the third-rail diamonds. The balls aren't on track 3.0, but they are close. Paralleling from track 3.0 will reveal that 2.7 is the proper track to use in your calculations.

The next step is to find the line of aim for the cueball.

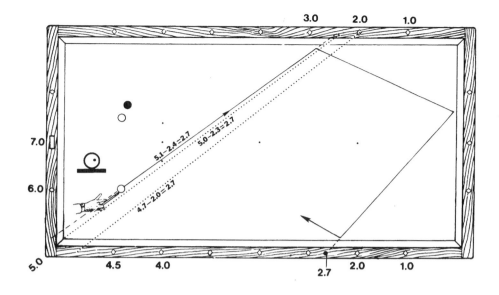

65 Applying the formula

Continuing the example begun in the last diagram, stand behind the 5.0 corner and look for a first-rail number that when subtracted from the cueball origin will equal 2.7. If you point your cue toward 2.0, the butt would have to cross 4.7 to provide a difference of 2.7. Laying the butt across the corner and mentally subtracting 2.7 from 5.0 gives a first-rail aiming point of 2.3. This last trial run gives a line that almost passes through the cueball. Parallel over to the cueball and you have a cueball origin of 5.1 and a first-rail aiming point of 2.4. Shoot with running English and the cueball will go into 2.7 on the third rail and from there to the score. It's like shooting fish in a barrel.

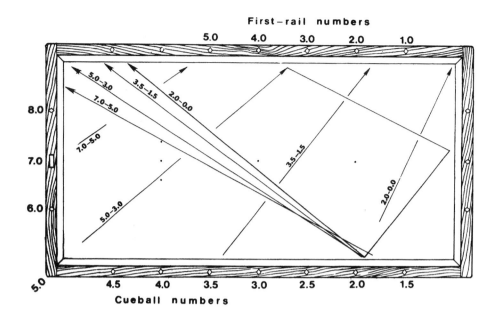

First-rail numbers

5.0   4.0   3.0   2.0   1.0

8.0

7.0

6.0

5.0

4.5   4.0   3.5   3.0   2.5   2.0   1.5

Cueball numbers

66 Track shifts

Unfortunately, the tracks given in Diagram 63 are good only for a cueball starting from the corner or close to it. The tracks cross the table at slightly different angles when the cueball starts from other places. The phenomenon will here be called track shifts. On your own table, shoot a cueball with running English and moderate speed from 7.0 to 5.0, from 5.0 to 3.0, from 3.5 to 1.5, and from 2.0 to 0.0 (the last requires a little extra English). You'll reach 2.0 on the third rail in each case but different points on the fourth rail, as shown in this diagram. Memorizing track 2.0 fourth-rail termination points for every possible cueball origin is too much to ask even of the most fanatic. It's enough to know the 7.0–5.0 and the 2.0–0.0 paths—others can be approximated from those known lines.

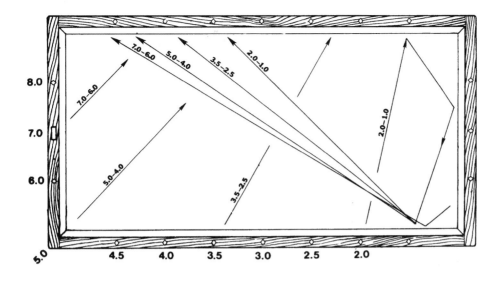

67 More track shifts

Here is how track 1.0 shifts for various cueball starting points. Memorize the 7.0–6.0 and the 2.0–1.0 paths and the rest can be fairly closely guessed when the need arises. Frank Torres, the 1974 and 1978 United States champion, urged me to warn you that when shooting from cueball numbers higher than 7.0, the contact point on the third rail is closer to the lower right corner than the system predicts.

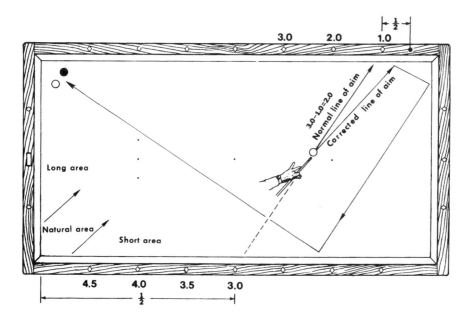

68 The Seattle Kid's allowances

Seventy years ago or so, The Seattle Kid, a.k.a. Arthur Kreshell, devised a method of compensating for track shifts when the player is trying to reach fourth-rail target points. The Kid used the "normal" tracks given in Diagram 63 and applied various allowances when the cueball wasn't starting from the "natural area" in the corner.

To the right of the corner, the "short area," an amount must be deducted from the first-rail number found by the diamond-system formula; the amount grows with the distance of the cueball origin from the corner. Along the end rail, the "long area," an amount must be added to the first-rail number. In the diagram above, the object balls are in the corner. The normal track that runs into the corner is 2.0. The formula is satisfied by aiming at 1.0 on the first rail because the cueball number is then 3.0, a difference of 2.0. But as you learned from Diagram 66, track 2.0 doesn't run to the corner when the cueball number is 3.0. A correction is needed. What The Kid suggested is this: Whatever the ratio is of the distance of the cueball number from the corner to the length of the rail is the amount of the needed correction, in diamonds. That sounds complicated but is simple. In the diagram, the cueball number is 3.0, which is halfway along the side rail from the corner. The correction, therefore, is half a diamond, applied as shown. If the cueball number was 4.0, you would be only a quarter of the way up the length of the rail and the deduction would be a quarter of a diamond, and so on.

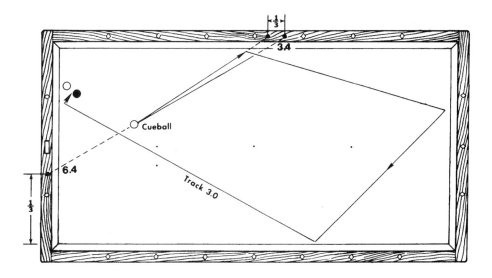

69 End-rail allowances

In The Seattle Kid's system of allowances, shooting from the end rail (the "long area") requires an addition to the first-rail number if you want to reach the same point on the fourth rail as a normal track. Normal track 3.0 in Diagram 63 will score the point given in the diagram. Aiming the cueball at 3.4 gives a cueball number of 6.4 and the desired difference of 3.0, but since the cueball is starting from a point that is roughly a third of the way along the end rail, a correction of a third of a diamond is made on the first rail.

In practice, I find that hardly any allowance is needed in the "long area" for angles of approach to the first rail of greater than about 30 degrees, unless the cloth is new.

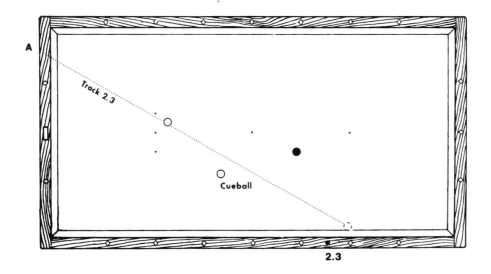

2.3

70 Using the system off a ball

The system can take some of the guesswork out of ball-first shots as well as banks. Let's say you have decided to play the diagrammed shot off the left side of the red ball and you would like to have a target on the first rail at which to carom the cueball. First, stand at A and find out what normal track the white ball is on. The dotted line shows that track 2.3 is about right.

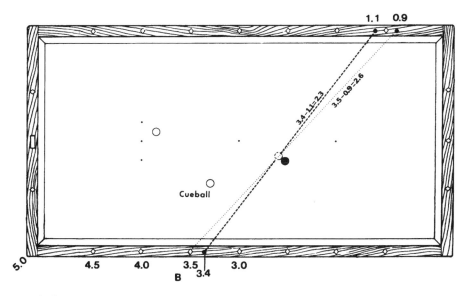

71 Trial runs

Continuing the example, the next step is to stand at B and find a first-rail aiming point that when subtracted from the cueball origin will equal 2.3. Using your cue if you like as a guide for your eye, sight along the left edge of the red, which is the line the cueball will take off the red. From cueball number 3.5, a line that passes the left edge of the red terminates at 0.9 on the first rail for a difference of 2.6, which is too large. Pivoting your cue slowly with the red ball as a fulcrum, you will eventually find two numbers that are 2.3 apart, in this example 3.4 and 1.1. Now a correction must be made because the cueball isn't starting from the corner.

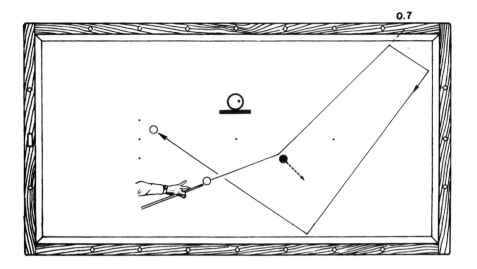

72 Applying the allowance

Continuing the example, there remains the matter of applying an appropriate allowance. The cueball number found in the last diagram is 3.4, which is roughly four-tenths of the way along the side rail from the corner. The correction, therefore, is four-tenths of a diamond, making the proper aiming point 0.7. If you can carom the cueball into 0.7 on the first rail with running English, you'll make the shot or come awfully close to it.

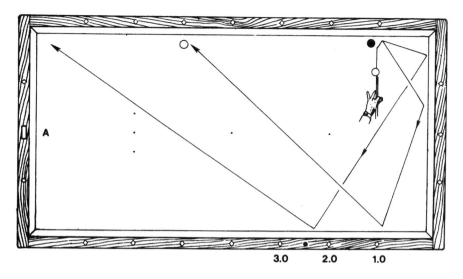

3.0   2.0   1.0

73 Two priceless short-angle tracks

Knowing these two tracks comes in handy in almost every game. When the cue-ball number is less than, say, 3.5, a third-rail return of 1.0 connects with the third diamond from the corner on the fourth rail. In the diagram, the path is shown scoring a point—by extension, the point would also score if the white ball were at A. A return of 2.5 on the third rail connects with the diagonally opposite corner. Knowing just one short-angle track, say the 1.0 track drawn here, enables you to estimate others, for a difference of half a diamond on the third rail results in a difference of a whole diamond on the fourth rail.

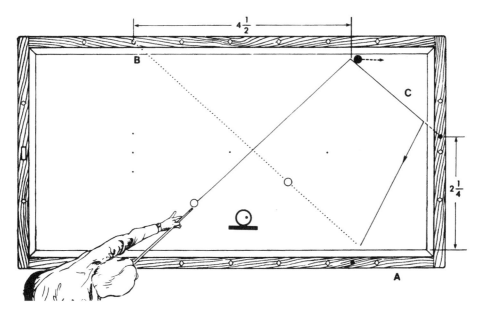

74 The Rodriguez Legacy

An old man, now forty years dead, passed along to me a handy second-rail system. Where Ernie Rodriguez learned it, I don't know. In the diagram, the first object ball is on the rail, which means that the contact point for the cueball on the first rail is fixed. Because speed on natural shots should always be between soft and moderate, the only variable the player has left to work with is English. The more right English is used, the farther up the third rail the cueball can be sent, within limits. In laying out this shot in your mind, it would help to know where the cueball must hit the second rail, and that's what the Rodriguez Legacy provides. First, the proper scoring track from the third to the fourth rails must be estimated by standing at A and applying the knowledge you have absorbed from the previous diagram. The correct track, let us say, is 1.5, which terminates on the fourth rail at B. Measure the distance from B to the first-rail contact point, which is $4\frac{1}{2}$ diamonds in this example. Half of that amount, $2\frac{1}{4}$ diamonds, measured in diamonds from the near corner, determines the second-rail contact point.

Ernie told me one other thing before he died. If the cueball is at C, spin draw must be used to bring the cueball off the red. In that case a half-diamond must be added to the calculated point on the second rail.

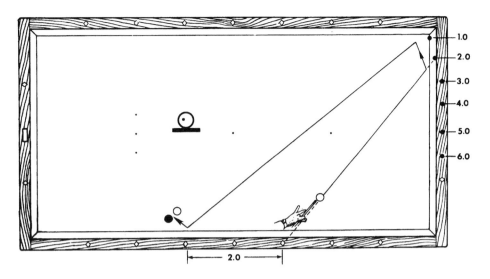

75 The dreaded "plus" system

I call the so-called plus system "dreaded" because it is so sensitive to slight changes in English and speed. Still, it's better than nothing for shots requiring the cueball to be angled into the end rail and you had better add it to your repertoire. In the plus system the end rail is numbered as shown. If you shoot straight at the 4.0 spot (not at the point on the edge of the rubber opposite it) with running English, the cueball will return to the lower rail four diamonds farther down than the point of cueball origin.

Diagrammed is a shot in which the object balls are two diamonds away from the cueball along the rail. To make the shot, the player aims at point 2.0 on the end rail.

Warning: When the cueball approaches the end rail at less than a 30-degree angle, the plus system works poorly or not at all. Resort to judgment there.

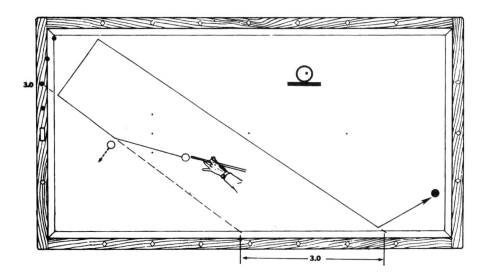

76 The plus system off a ball

Using the plus system off a ball requires estimating where the cueball must hit the third rail to make the point, then counting the diamonds to the point of cueball origin. The line of sight to the first rail runs from the side of the first ball. You may have to aim at several points before finding two numbers that match.

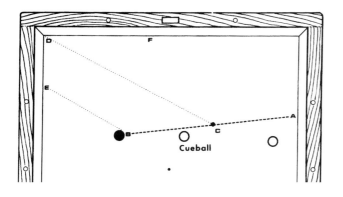

77 No-English parallel system

This shot can be made by going off the right side of the red without English to point E, then F, then to A. The angle of the line BE can be found by a simple parallel system. First, estimate the required contact point on the third rail, A. Imagine a line AB and its midpoint, C. Project a line from C to the corner, D. BE is parallel to CD.

The system can be helpful in laying out long-angle no-English patterns, too, like the one in Diagram 29. Always start by estimating the third-rail contact point and imagining a line from there to the first ball.

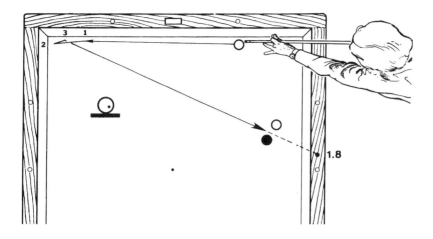

78 A system for doubling the rail

Place the cueball close to the end rail, shoot softly with maximum reverse English, double the rail, and see how far from the corner the cueball returns to the fourth rail. On some tables it is possible to reach the second diamond, on others only a diamond and a half. I will assume for the sake of illustration that on your table you can reach 1.8. Your double-the-rail maximum, therefore, is 1.8 and the diagrammed shot can be made.

If the object balls weren't so far from the end rail, you wouldn't have to use maximum English.

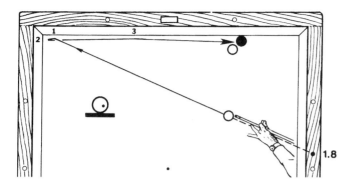

79 Double-the-rail maximum

If 1.8 is your double-the-rail maximum (see previous diagram), then you can also double the rail by shooting *out of* 1.8. The shot portrayed here is just barely possible, provided you shoot softly, use extreme right English, and aim slightly left of the corner, relying on curve to make the cueball hit the end rail first. If the cueball was even an inch farther from the end rail, you would know that the shot is impossible.

(As a practical matter it is advisable to take a tenth off your maximum when running the pattern in this direction. The curve of the cueball path as it approaches the corner means that in effect the origin is slightly higher than 1.8.)

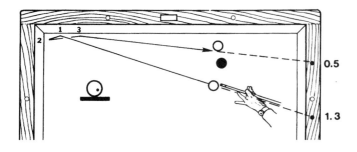

80 Components of the maximum

The last two diagrams lead up to this rule: On extreme English double-the-rail shots, the cueball origin and the fourth-rail return always add up to the predetermined maximum. The shot in the diagram above can be made because 1.3 plus 0.5 equals 1.8. If either the cueball or the object balls are farther from the end rail, the shot is impossible.

When the shot involves components that add up to less than your maximum, use less English. How much less? That's for you to find out.

5

extensions, variations,
extremes, and guidelines

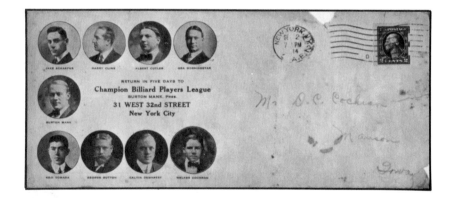

(Byrne Collection)

Because the balls never stop in precisely the same places twice, every pattern in the diagrams can be used for an infinite number of shots. And every pattern has a mirror image, an extension to additional rails, and variations in which the cueball path is distorted by spin or speed. Thus the reader who has been paying attention is already in possession of a formidable arsenal of offensive weapons. In this section we will discuss a variety of shots and ideas that more or less follow from the material already presented. Then we'll be ready for some really interesting stuff!

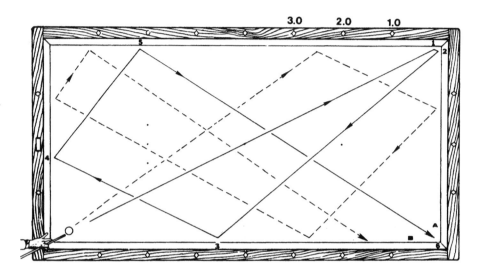

81 Twice around from the corner

A good way to test an unfamiliar table is to bank the cueball "twice around" with running English. If it follows the solid line off the fifth rail and enters squarely into the low right corner, the table is "true," and the same can be said for your stroke, speed, and English. (I will assume from here on that your technique is impeccable.) If the cueball hits A on the sixth rail, as it will on new imported cloth, the table is "long." B as a termination point means the table is "short." Once you know how a table rolls, you can make appropriate aiming adjustments.

It is worth the small effort involved to memorize the two paths given in this diagram as they will prove useful in planning many twice-around banks.

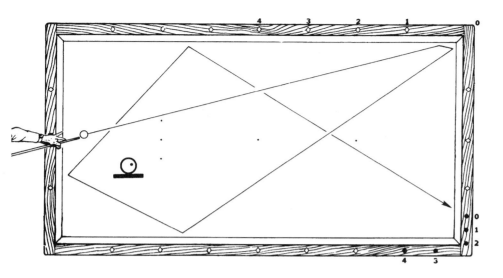

82 Twice around from the nameplate

Here's another useful pattern to burn into your mind. Note that the first-rail diamonds are numbered. Shooting from the nameplate into any of those numbers will send the cueball to the matching number on the sixth rail.

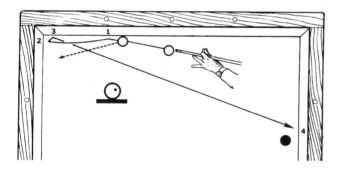

83 Smash-through extended

If you can make the shot in Diagram 20, try this extension of the same idea. Considerable force and accuracy are needed, but the shot is quite practical on fast cloth.

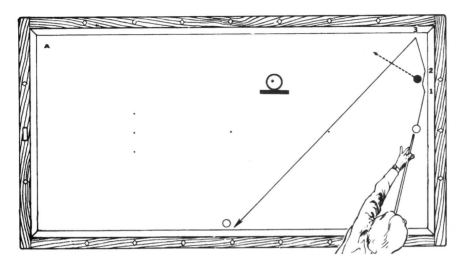

84 Ticky extended

When the first ball is close to the rail, a ticky (Diagram 39) can be extended with considerable accuracy. The second ball could be at A, a further extension requiring extra speed. Down through the corridors of time, novices have tended not to notice extended tickys. Maybe they will now.

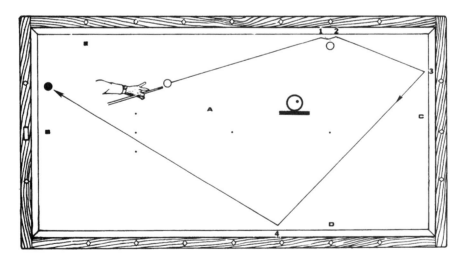

85 Another ticky extended

Here the ticky extended is the easiest of several options. Extend it farther for a red ball at E or A. Use less English for a red ball at B. Draw off the first rail will pull the cueball to C and D.

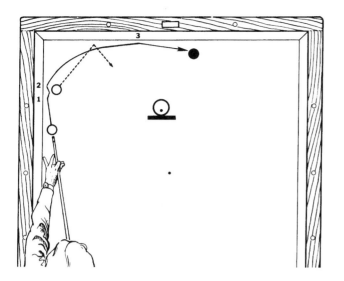

86 Ticky bent by draw

Not easy, but not particularly tough, either. The red ball can be all the way over by the right corner. Use plenty of draw and don't shoot hard. The shot becomes much more difficult when the cueball and first ball aren't so close to the rail. If you are trying it for the first time, put the white a ball-width from the rail and the cueball a half-ball-width.

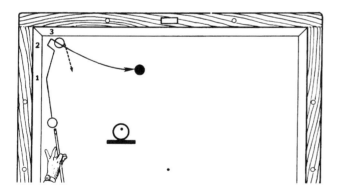

87 Ticky bent by follow

A ticky can be distorted by follow if the first ball is in the corner. The shot can be a lifesaver when your opponent has left you at the opposite end of the table and when all other options would require divine intervention.

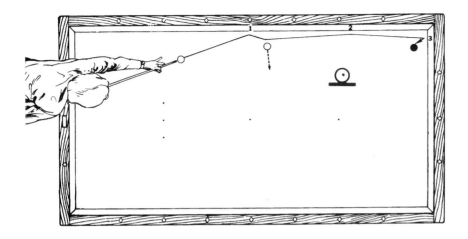

88 Soft ticky

When the first ball is close to the rail and you want the cueball to stay close to the rail in the ticky pattern, shoot as softly as possible and use hardly any English. When the first ball is less than a ball-width from the rail, there is no way to keep the cueball from springing away except by the hard-to-judge follow ticky (Diagram 159).

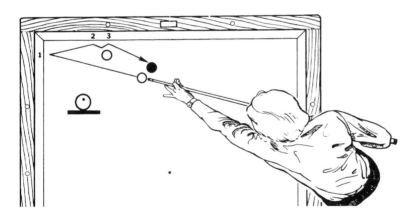

89 Snap-away back-up ticky

The danger with a back-up ticky (Diagram 41) like this is that the cueball will go through the gaping hole between the red and the rail. To offset that possibility, use high English and firm speed and try to get a full hit on the white off the second rail. In cases even more severe than this, it is necessary to add a touch of hold-up and hit the first rail closer to the corner.

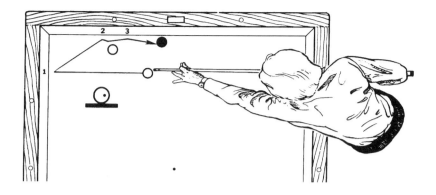

90 Angled ticky

The problem here is just the opposite of the one in the previous diagram. The red is so close to the rail that the cueball might miss it by springing too sharply off the third rail. The solution is to approach the second rail at a steeper angle with the aid of right English. It takes getting used to.

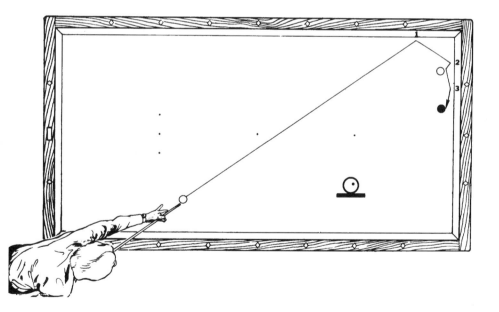

91 Diagonal back-up ticky

When your opponent thinks he has left you safe, it feels good to pull off this shot, which isn't difficult in the given position.

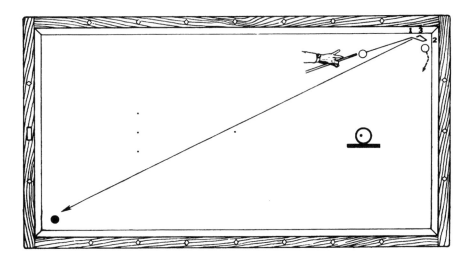

92 Spin-out extended

Nothing more than a long version of Diagram 44, with a smaller margin of error.

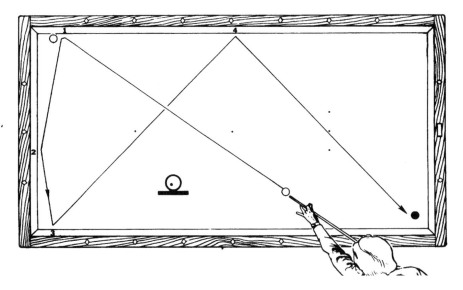

93 Rail-first short angle extended

A long version of Diagram 49 that comes up every hundred points or so. Remember that the second ball can be anywhere along the path that the cueball takes off the third and fourth rails.

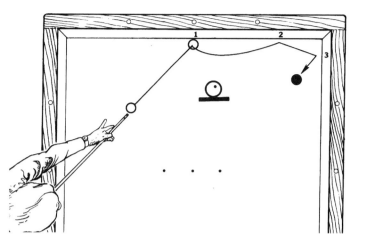

94 Smash-through back to the rail

Fairly common. Be sure to hit the cueball extremely high. An interesting strobe-light photo of this shot is given in Willie Hoppe's *Billiards As It Should Be Played,* page 55.

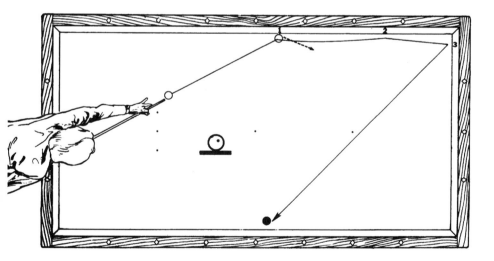

95 Long-range smash-through

The best shot under the circumstances. It sometimes scores without the cueball getting back to the side rail; if it *does* get back, as in the diagram, the red is a big ball.

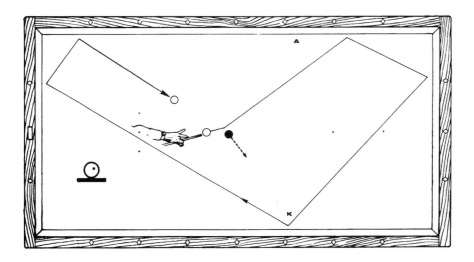

96 Five-rail option off a ball

Beginners are forever trying to make this shot three rails by drawing the cueball to A. Five rails as diagrammed is much easier because all that is needed is normal speed and English. To avoid a heartbreaking kiss, make sure to hit enough of the red so that it is beyond point K before the cueball arrives there.

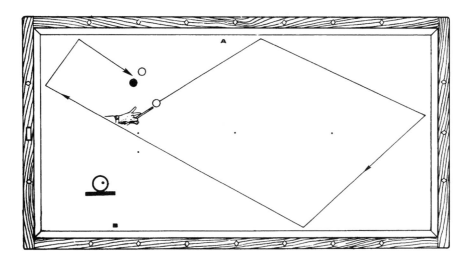

97 Five-rail bank option

This shot can be made three rails first by shooting toward A or B. You can either learn from experience or from me that the five-rail path is easiest to judge. (Track 3.0 is quite predictable.)

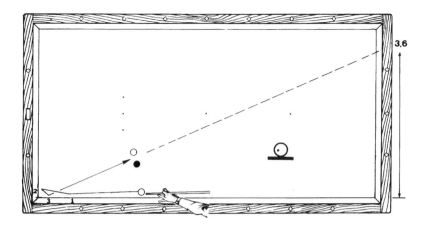

98 Doubling the long rail

If you can hit 1.8 the short way (Diagram 78), you can hit 3.6 the long way. The path drawn here, therefore, is feasible.

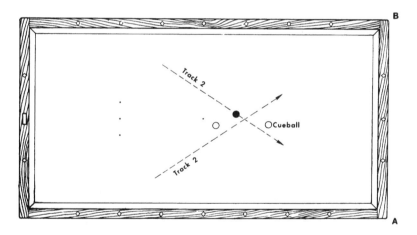

99 The "two-line" subtlety

For revealing secrets like this, I am putting myself in danger of becoming known as "Old Blabbermouth." Look at the diagram. The shot can be made with natural English off either side of the white. Which is best? By standing at A you can see that the red is on track 2.0, which leads to the corner on "normal" patterns (Diagram 63). From B you can see that the red is not quite on the 2.0 track that comes off the other long rail. The path leading to B is best for this shot because if the cueball misses the red going in, it might get it coming out. In a sense, the red is a big ball going into the B corner but not going into the A corner. See next diagram.

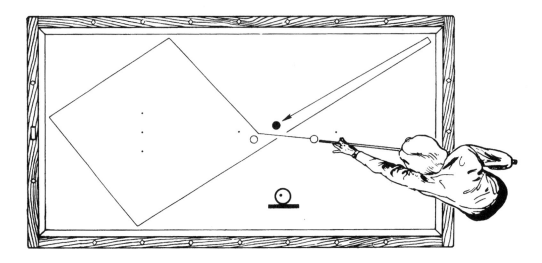

100 The two-line applied

To "lock up" this shot, the shooter plays it a hair long (toward the short-rail side of the corner) so that if the cueball misses the red off the third rail it will hit it off the fifth, as diagrammed. If the red was an inch or two on the other side of the two-line, the shot should be played a hair short so that if the cueball misses the red going in, it might make it by "backing out" of the corner.

Don't try to employ the principle of the two-line when the second ball is, say, six inches to one side or the other. Then you must make a definite decision on whether to play it three rails or five. (Five usually gives better position for the following shot.)

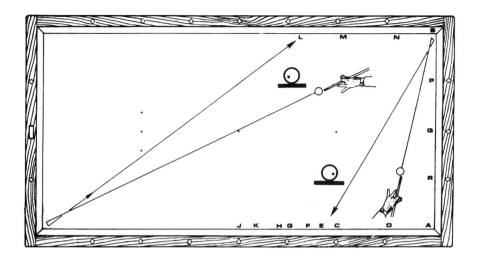

101 Short-angle and plus system extremes

Here's a handy grab bag of extreme-English paths. Shooting from A to B with maximum right springs the cueball to C. D to B (as drawn) returns to E. C to B returns to F. G to B returns to H. From the middle of the long rail you can no longer get to the point of cueball origin by shooting into the corner. J to B returns only to K. The paths are handy because the plus system (Diagram 75) doesn't work for these into-the-corner angles.

Some unlikely shots can be made by overloading the plus system with extreme English on long diagonal patterns. Shooting out of B, for example, toward the lower left corner, returns the cueball to L. P returns to M, Q to N, and R to B.

Your stroke and your table will no doubt yield somewhat different results.

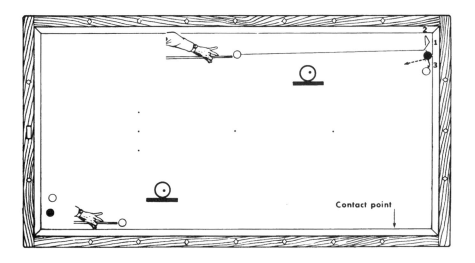

Contact point

102 The tight snake shot

When playing a snake shot (Diagram 21) like the one shown here in the upper right corner, in which there is little room to maneuver, the secret is to shoot as softly as the required action will permit. Too much speed sends the cueball into the second rail before it has had a chance to bend.

Aiming a long double-the-rail

On three-rail-first, double-the-rail shots, use a contact point fairly close to the corner to minimize the amount of English needed.

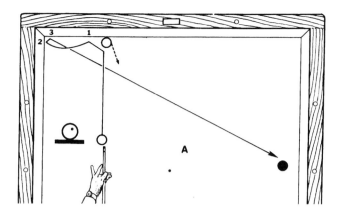

103 Snake shot extended

Double-the-rail maximums can be exceeded on snake shots because of the way follow changes the cueball's angle of approach to the second rail. If 1.8 is your
double-the-rail maximum (Diagram 78), then 2.0 or even 2.5 can be reached with
the pattern given here. The shot diagrammed can't be made from A because not
as much bend can be induced.

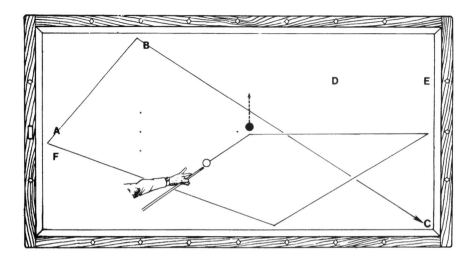

104 End-rail right-angle maximum

Going off a ball into the center of the end rail at right angles with maximum right English sends the cueball along the path diagrammed here. The second ball can be at A, B, C, or intermediate points. The path is practically the same when shooting directly into the rail (not off a ball). Shifting the approach line one diamond in either direction changes the third-rail contact point about a half a diamond. Thus, D to E sends the cueball to the third rail behind F.

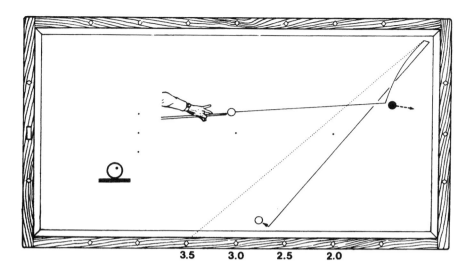

| 3.5 | 3.0 | 2.5 | 2.0 |

105 Stretching with follow

At first glance it might seem that the shot off the left side of the red is impossible. Applying the diamond system suggests that since the cueball origin is 2.5, the cueball will return to a point two-and-a-half diamonds from the corner on the third rail, a full diamond short of the second ball. With follow, however, the cueball path bends on the way to the corner and the effective cueball origin number is 3.5. Making use of this curve is called stretching a shot.

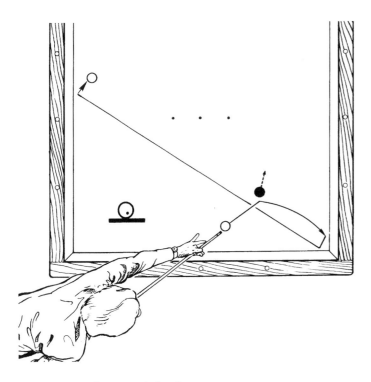

106 Stretching with draw

Straight-line draw to the corner with deadball or stun action (see Diagram 43 in Book One) isn't sufficient here. The cueball must be made to curve on its way to the first rail to create the proper angle of approach. For a "spread" draw, as it is called, rather than a deadball draw, hit the cueball lower and the object ball thinner.

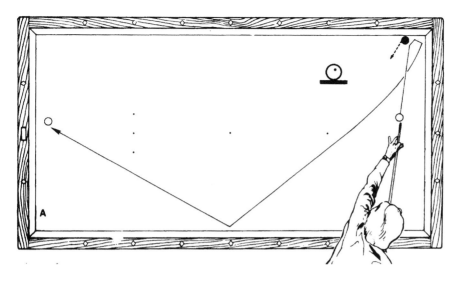

107 Second-rail stretch

In Diagram 12 it was shown that shooting with follow into a ball on the rail makes the cueball bend on its way to the second rail. Here the object ball is so close to both the first and second rails that the bend doesn't have time to occur until the cueball is on its way to the third rail. The cueball by means of this action can even be sent to the corner at A, though to reach there it helps to use a hair of left English as well as follow.

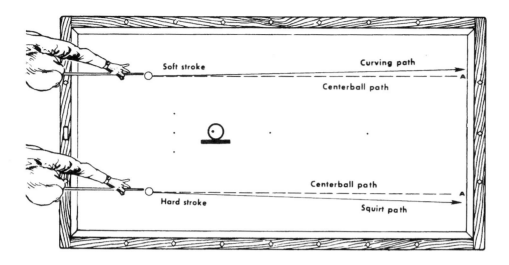

108 Curve versus "squirt"

"Squirt" might be the reason you miss length-of-the-table shots that must be struck hard with maximum English. If you shoot with left English and softly enough to permit the spin to work against the cloth as the ball rolls down the table, it will curve in the direction of the English . . . unless your cue is exactly level, in which case there can be no cueball curve.

But even with a level cue, if you shoot more firmly, the cueball will diverge along a line opposite the English, as shown in the diagram. I call this phenomenon squirt; others call it deflection. If you shoot hard with maximum sidespin, squirt can deflect the cueball path two inches or more over the length of the table.

6

fifteen draw, spin, time, and kiss-back shots

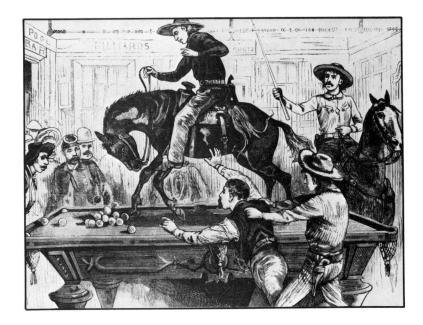

Texans horsing around.
(*Illustrated Police News*, 1888)

Here we have the pickles and relish of billiards, the tricky and ingenious stratagems that are a measure of a player's imagination and knowledge of the game.
Don't pay too much attention to the exact placement of the balls in the diagrams.
Pay attention instead to the *ideas,* which are applicable to an infinite number of
shots.

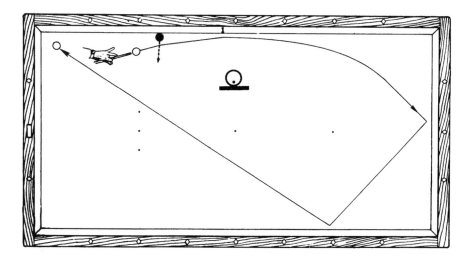

109 Thin-hit side-rail draw

The white ball is big in the corner and there seems to be no way to make use of
it. There is a way, though. Hit the red extremely thin . . . just tickle it . . . and use
low draw. The path will bend as shown. The shot requires finesse, not power.
Without draw you'll miss by three feet.

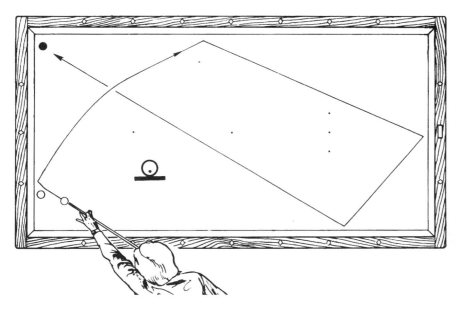

110 Thin-hit end-rail draw

Another application of drawing off a ball that is close to a rail. Use no English, just draw.

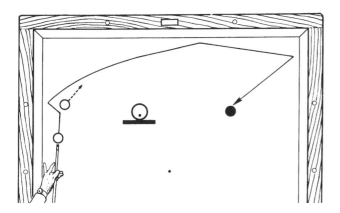

111 Short-angle draw

Don't baby this one—it must be struck crisply.

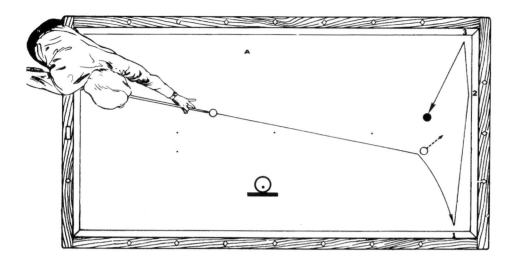

112 Cut short-angle draw

Trying to deadball the cueball to the side rail on this short-angle shot will likely bank the white off one rail into the red. To miss the kiss you must cut the white more and compensate with draw. From point A, deadball action can be used because the kiss can be missed driving the white at right angles into the end rail. (Compare Hoppe's Diagram number 69.)

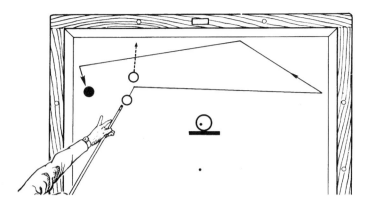

113 Short-angle spin shot

The spin shot is beautiful to watch when executed with control. By hitting an object ball full, you can make the cueball travel slowly across the table while spinning like a top. It gains speed each time it hits a rail. The technique is used to create angles for scoring that don't seem to be there, and to enlarge the final target when the second ball is frozen or close to the third rail. Most spin shots must be hit fairly hard to make sure they are still spinning when they reach the third rail. (See also Diagram 3.)

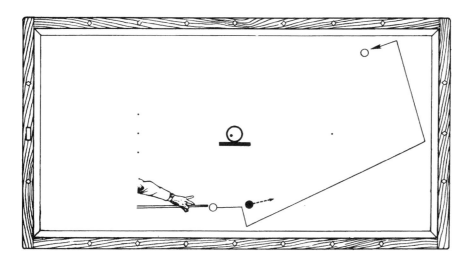

114 Long-angle spin shot

Hit the red ball full and fairly hard, which removes most of the speed from the cueball but hardly any of the English. In aiming a shot like this where the first ball is close to a rail, pick out a contact point on the second rail, keeping in mind that the cueball will arrive there with tremendous spin.

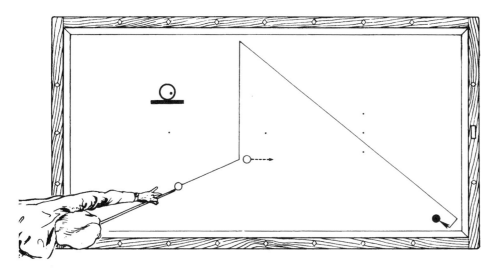

115 Another long-angle spin shot

A spin shot is used here to avoid cutting the white directly into the red.

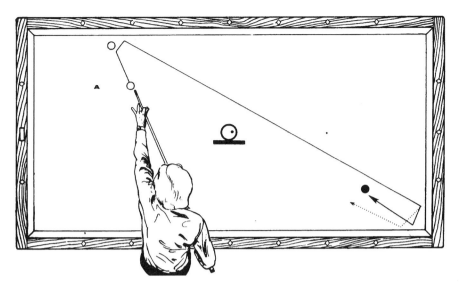

116 Draw-back spin shot

The diagrammed shot might not seem feasible, but because the white ball can be hit full, the cueball can be sent slowly into the corner with lots of spin and will spurt sharply off the second rail into a scoring angle. From A the shot is impossible, because when the first ball is hit thin, the cueball enters the corner with too much speed in relation to its spin and will follow the dotted line.

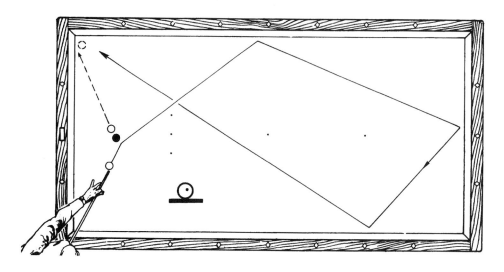

117 An easy time shot

A time shot is one in which the shooter deliberately puts all three balls in motion. The time shot in the diagram is a much higher percentage shot than the bank. Wait and watch for opportunities like this.

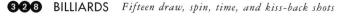

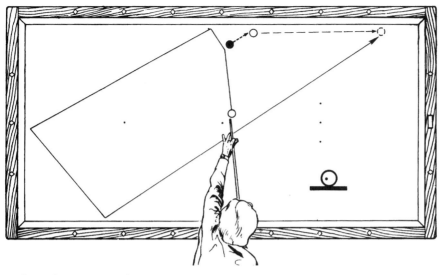

118 A harder time shot

I made this time shot in a 1977 tournament game against Sudden Sam Worley of Simi Valley, California. It's harder than the previous one because the red has to be driven into the white with more accuracy. In aiming, first fix in your mind the necessary speed and cut, then adjust the English to send the cueball off the first rail at the right angle.

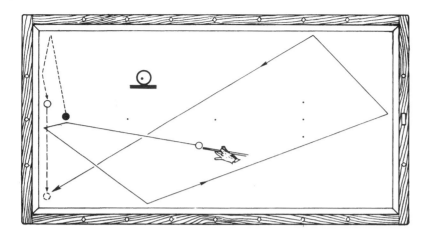

119 A very hard time shot

This is murder, but on rare occasions it is the only shot that has any reasonable chance of scoring. Something quite similar is diagrammed in *Championship Billiards Old and New* by John A. Thatcher, published in 1898, where I learned that the idea was once tried by a certain professor, Louis Reed. After striking the cueball, the professor in his excitement took several backward steps and fell out of a window. According to Thatcher, he managed to climb back in in time to cry, "It's going to count, by gosh!"

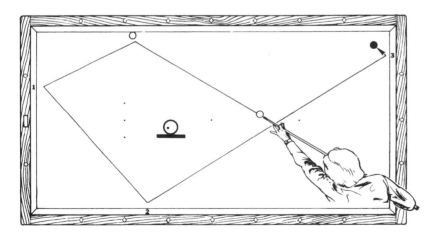

120 Side-rail kiss-back to the end rail

A good idea to file away somewhere for use when everything else looks worse.

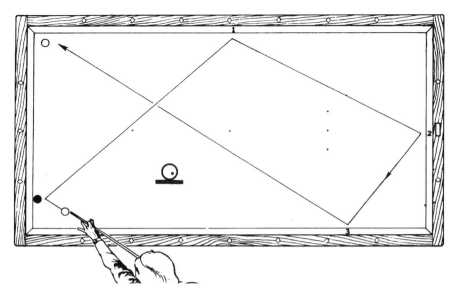

121 End-rail kiss-back

When the Diagram 110 path is too much to ask for, a kiss-back comes into consideration.

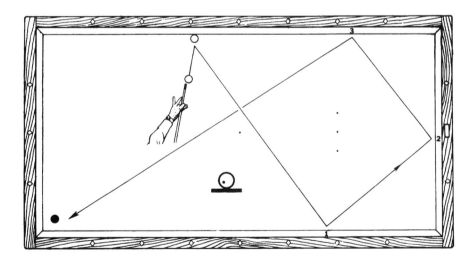

122 Side-rail kiss-back

An often overlooked pattern. Always hit the cueball below center when kissing back off a ball. Note that left English is needed to make the cueball run around the table naturally after hitting the first rail.

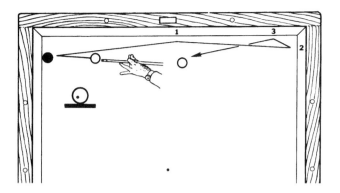

123 Kiss-back through the hole

I thought of this pattern one morning while lying in bed staring at the ceiling. When it finally came up in a game about a year later, I pounced on it with almost undignified alacrity.

playing safe, ducking kisses, and getting position

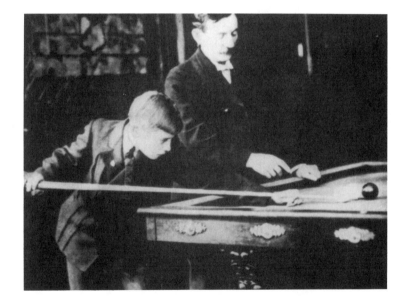

7

Jacob "The Wizard" Schaefer, the world's best player at the turn of the century, instructs his son Jake Junior in about 1908. Young Jake took the world title from Willie Hoppe in 1921 at the age of twenty-seven and is still regarded as the greatest balkline artist in history.
(Byrne Collection)

This section and the next cover advanced strategy and tactics . . . and by "advanced" I don't necessarily mean difficult. Setting yourself up for an easy shot, for example, is often merely a matter of being aware of a few principles.

The games of many American players are disfigured by an excessive concern for safety. They concentrate so hard on leaving the balls tough for their opponents that they often fail to make shots that are relatively easy, and they shrink from taking the chances that high runs are made of. Safety players can be hard to beat, though, at least in time to get home at a decent hour.

Not that you should ignore defense. You'll be chopped up by good players if you do. You must learn to select the shot and the cueball speed that will protect you in case of a miss, particularly on low-percentage shots. Forget safety on big-ball shots and naturals and devote all of your attention to scoring and perhaps a little to playing position. After all, even if you miss, the balls might end up in difficult positions. Studying the world's best players for almost forty years has convinced me that on the great majority of shots offense is the best defense. Out*score* the other guy and you'll win.

It's easy to play safe. All you have to do is leave the other cueball far from the object balls, ideally at the other end of the table. Your opponent won't be much of a threat if he has to cross nine or ten feet of green before he can even hit a ball. The rule of thumb for safety play is: "Easy up to the red, hard away from the white." In other words, shoot softly when you are trying to score on the red so that the cueball will remain near it if you miss while the opponent's cueball, presumably, goes elsewhere. When trying to score on the white, shoot hard enough to get your ball far from his if you miss. Not all shots permit you this luxury.

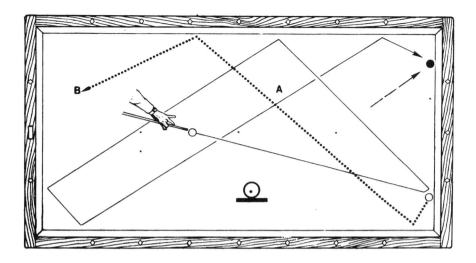

124 A choice of shots

In this symmetrical position there are four- and five-rail shots off either object ball. In choosing between them, several safety considerations arise. When your opponent's cueball is stuck on a rail, it can be argued that it should be left there on the grounds that he will be limited in the kinds of English he can apply. But shooting five rails off the right side of red, using a mirror image of the diagrammed path, you would leave your cueball near his in case of a miss, a violation of the safety principle that calls for leaving your opponent's cueball in as much isolation as possible.

Best is to play off the white, as shown. Your cueball will "die" near the red, and his will be sent at least five feet down the table. One last point: Should you try to score off four rails (dashed arrow) by hitting the white thin, or five rails as drawn? Thin might leave the white near A, not far from your cueball if you miss and it rebounds a couple of feet from the end rail. The five-rail option requires a fuller hit and sends the white farther down the table, to the vicinity of B.

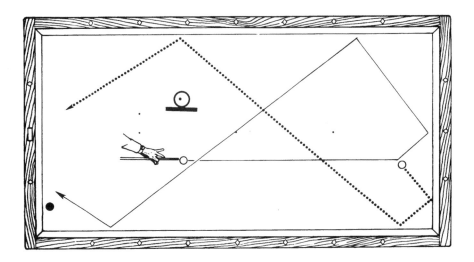

125 A typical sellout

When your opponent needs only a few points and you need fifteen, you must do your best to keep him from getting anything too easy. Don't play this shot as diagrammed because the three balls end up in the same part of the table. See next diagram.

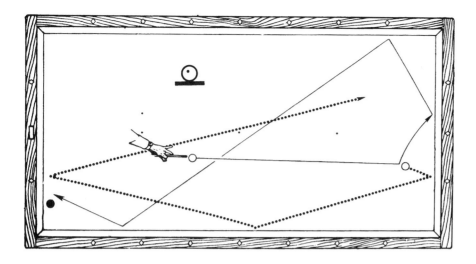

126 Avoiding a sellout

This is the previous shot played a safer way. Use more follow and hit the white fuller, driving it down the table and back to the other end. Now if you miss, your hated rival is far from his work. The idea is one of many I've been given by Al Gilbert of Hollywood, California, seven times United States champion, who retired from tournament play in 1993.

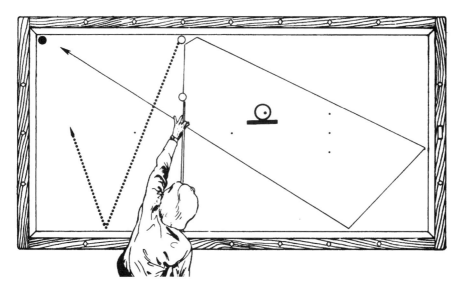

127 False safety

Players who spend their lives shooting easy to the red and hard to the white some-times do so even when it makes no sense, as in this case. The white is going to stay at the left end of the table anyway, so the cueball might as well be stroked with some authority to avoid drifts and roll-offs. There is a second reason for using speed in the diagrammed shot and that is to try to relocate the red ball if you score. Not only is a ball that deep in the corner a small target, it usually can't be used as the first ball, which reduces your options.

Easy-up-the-red players hurt themselves in other ways as well. They some-times miss shots by not shooting quite hard enough, which never happens to more freewheeling shooters, and they often leave their cueball so close to the red when they miss that they leave a good bank. Moral: When you decide to play easy up to the red, use enough speed to get a foot or two past it if you miss.

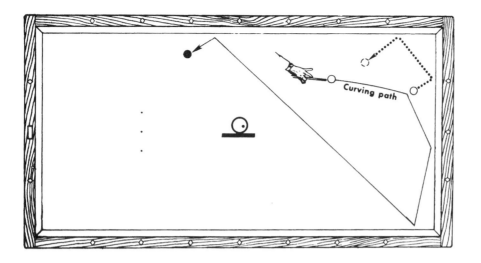

Curving path

128 Finesse safety

Using the plus system (Diagram 75) here poses a problem from a defensive point of view because the white ball will be banked down the table to join the fun . . . and possibly spoil the fun with a kiss. To keep the white ball from traveling very far, use extreme right English, shoot softly, allow for the curve, and hit the white thin. The required "touch" will come to you in time.

A new look at old shots

Now that you've been exposed to defensive thinking, we can look more deeply into some shots previously discussed.

Diagram 4—Cut the red at right angles to the side rail to keep it at the left end of the table, and use enough speed to get away from the white if you miss. If colors are reversed, shoot softly to die near the second ball. The same advice applies to Diagram 5.

Diagram 7—Try not to hit the white so full that it will zigzag down the table to join the other two balls.

Diagram 23—There is a nice subtlety here when the object-ball colors are reversed. Try for the third rail at A because, if you miss, the cueball will still have running English and can more easily be made to roll far from the ball in the corner. Going for the pattern diagrammed is more dangerous from a safety point of view (when the ball in the corner is the white) because the cueball, if you miss, will hit the side rail and the next rail with hold-up English, which tends to kill speed.

Diagram 25—Shoot hard enough to return the cueball to the left end of the table and cut the red thinly enough to keep it there.

Diagram 34—The thin hit, as drawn, is better than a full hit because the opponent's cueball is cut away from the final location of the other two balls.

Diagram 52—Shooting softly here in the interests of safety throws away an almost sure score. Many shots are harder to make if shot softly because they have little or no English left on the third rail. While the choice between "cinch speed" and "safe speed" is sometimes agonizing, there is no reason to hesitate when the second ball is big.

A word about kissing

Some players have an uncanny knack of seeing the possibility of kisses that are invisible to others. It might be a congenital gift that can't be taught, like the ability to yodel. As a teacher, all I can suggest for developing the knack is to try to profit from your mistakes. When you get a kiss, particularly of the resounding full-in-the-face variety, make a conscious effort to recall exactly how the balls were placed at the beginning so that you'll recognize the danger the next time.

When you know the shot has a kiss in it, you have to distort the pattern somehow or shoot something else. Often you can't tell for sure whether there is a kiss or not and you are faced with the choice of making the shot tougher by introducing distortion or playing it naturally and accepting the risk. You'll have to learn to weigh the odds yourself.

One of the most horrible things in the world is to make a fantastic hit on the first ball and be robbed of the point at the last instant by a kiss that not even God Himself could have foreseen. Just as bad is when your opponent makes a terrible hit and gets kissed *into* the point. These things put a severe strain on the human personality. As Deadpan Dan McGoorty said, "A three-cushion player doesn't have to be married. He already has enough aggravation."

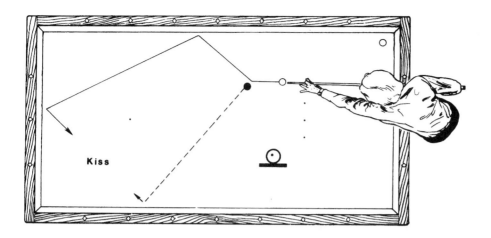

129 Natural kiss-out

An advantage of knowing the diamond system is that it often helps reveal kiss possibilities. On this shot, for example, the system teaches that on normal angles the cueball comes off the second diamond on the third rail on its way to the diagonally opposite corner. Since the line of travel for the object ball on cut shots is at right angles to the cueball's carom line off the object ball, it can be seen that there is a grave likelihood of disaster. Read on for what to do about it.

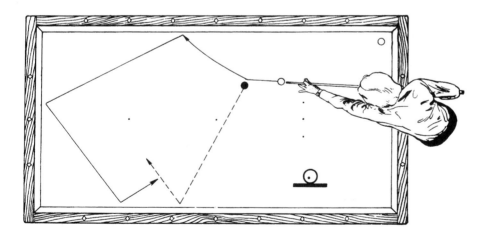

130 Ducking a kiss with draw

One way to miss the kiss is to cut the object ball away from the cueball's necessary contact point on the third rail. Draw bends the cueball back into a scoring path. Good players routinely use draw on this shot.

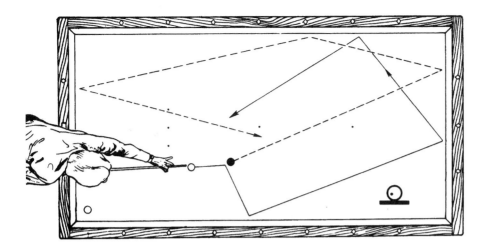

131 Ducking a kiss with drive

Another way to beat the kiss is to hit the object ball full, driving it as shown instead of cutting it. Don't drive the red into the end rail too close to the corner, though, or it might bank two rails into the white.

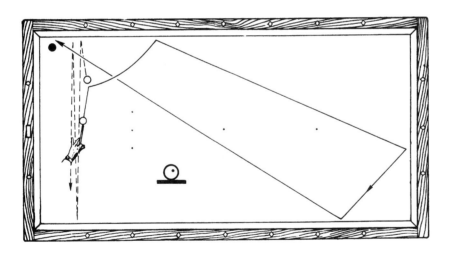

132 Ducking a kiss with follow

Cutting the white thin will send it directly into the red. Not quite so thin banks it twice across into the red. You must hit the white so full that it banks straight back and forth across the table. Hitting the cueball high and hard will bend it into a scoring path.

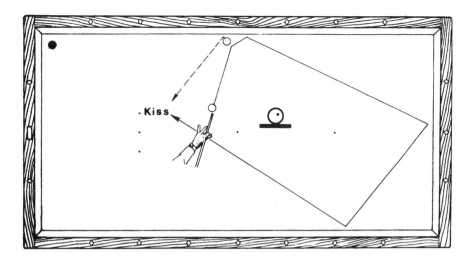

133 Another natural kiss-out

When the cueball and object-ball paths intersect and when it looks like they might arrive at the intersection at the same time, make a conscious decision to drive one ball or the other across the danger point first. In the diagrammed position the red ball is big, so liberties can be taken without too much risk of missing the shot. For instance, hitting a little more white ball will send it across the intersection well in advance of the cueball, while a touch of draw will bend the cueball back into the two-line.

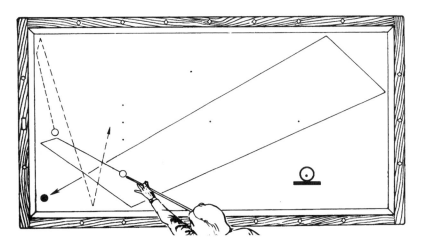

134 Missing the bank-across kiss

The easiest shot here is hitting the white thin with low left, but that banks the white into the red. To miss the kiss, hit more ball and use less English, making sure the white hits the end rail first. Because the white is hit fuller than it would be ordinarily on this pattern, more speed is needed to get the cueball around the table.

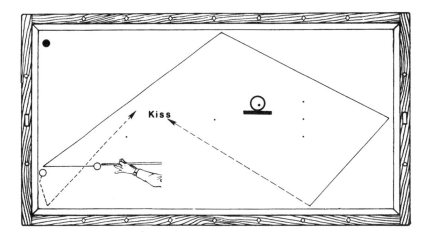

135 A four-rail kiss-out

There is a possible kiss on this common shot. You first must be aware of it, then you must do something about it if you think the prospect is ominous enough. Hitting more white ball will move the intersection farther to the right and, usually, will send the white across before the cueball arrives. A fuller hit can be compensated for with draw, as in Diagram 110.

Another new look at old shots

With kisses in mind, earlier diagrams can be reconsidered with profit. A sampling:

Diagram 1—Be careful not to bank the white into the red.

Diagram 2—Don't bank the white twice across into the red.

Diagram 3—A common error on this type of spin shot is to drive the red into the first rail near A, which sends it two rails into the white.

Diagram 8—The hit must be thin enough to keep the white from returning to the cueball path.

Diagram 15, right—Hit enough red ball to make sure it goes into the corner and back out before the white gets to the third rail.

Diagram 16, left—Sometimes, on patterns of this type, the first ball goes all the way up the table and back down into the second ball before the cueball gets there. Not all things in life are as we might wish them.

Diagram 23—It's depressing how often this shot is kissed out after the cueball leaves the third rail and seems headed happily home. At some angles (experience will tell you which ones) it is salubrious to hit the white ball thin with draw.

Diagram 24—As drawn, there is a big, fat kiss near the numeral 2. If the cueball was an inch or two to the right at the start, the first ball would be out of the way before the cueball gets to the second rail. If the kiss looks too ugly, you can always go back to the pattern given in Diagram 14, left.

On playing position

Attempting to leave the balls in good spots for a second shot is a practice that has generally been left to master players. Newcomers can't imagine how position can be played in a game apparently so abstract and formless. Many fairly good players never play position—they don't know the principles and they feel the first point is hard enough to make without worrying about the next one. Serendipity is their guide.

On many shots, however, as you will discover in the following sequence of diagrams, it is just as easy to play position as not. No extraordinary talent is required, just a little information. Part of what follows is based on my own ideas, part on my observations and discussions with top American players, and part on the pathbreaking work done on the subject by the world's foremost teacher of the game, René Vingerhoedt of Antwerp. During my visit to that Belgian city for the 1974 world's tournament, Vingerhoedt, world champion in 1948 and 1960, showed me the sketches he had made that illustrated in black and white what previously had existed only in the minds of the world's best players.

How do world champions like Belgium's Raymond Ceulemans and Sweden's Torbjorn Blomdahl compile tournament averages of 1.6, 1.8, and even 2.0 points per inning? How do they get so many runs of fifteen and more? Blomdahl is known for fantastic shotmaking, Ceulemans for speed control and defense; both are outstanding position players. We can't all have world-class strokes, touch, eyesight, nerves, discipline, and experience, but we can learn the principles of position play, which turn out to be not so difficult and mysterious.

The position player takes three approaches. Sometimes he tries to leave himself a specific type of shot, sometimes he tries to leave the balls in a way that will provide more than one option, and sometimes he simply tries to avoid leaving a ball or balls in unpromising positions. He sometimes misses a point because of his extra efforts, but if he is good enough, he is more than amply repaid with runs of points.

Some basics:

1. Don't land so softly on the second ball that you are hidden behind it. If you can only hit one ball, your options are greatly reduced.
2. It is usually best to be between the object balls.
3. When you can see that a certain speed will leave the balls in a tough position for your next shot, use more speed even though you can't predict the outcome.
4. Think twice about leaving a ball in the corner because in that position it usually can't be used as the first ball, thus reducing options.
5. Don't leave an object ball near the middle of an end rail.
6. Try not to leave the cueball facing the object balls with an end rail behind them; better to have the cueball between the short rail and the object balls.
7. When faced with a shot of average difficulty or easier, think about position rather than safety.
8. When faced with a choice of shots and speeds, take the course that will leave as many balls as possible in the central area of the table; there are bound to be several options, one of which may be ideal.
9. Trying to leave yourself a certain type of shot, as illustrated in most of the following diagrams, is generally feasible only when you can land gently on the second ball. If the cueball approaches the second ball with speed, there is no way to predict the outcome.
10. If you miss too many shots because you are trying to play position, cut back on position play.
11. Don't play position by attempting to hit the second object ball on one side or the other.

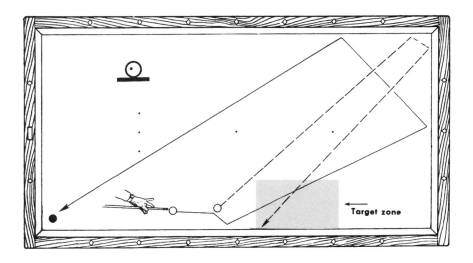

Target zone

136 Two-rail position cut

One of the easiest position patterns. In a 1977 exhibition game win over a three-time national champion, I used it five times in a run of eight points. All you have to do is make sure the first object ball hits the long rail first and comes to rest in the shaded area. If you land lightly on the red with the cueball you are almost bound to have another easy shot.

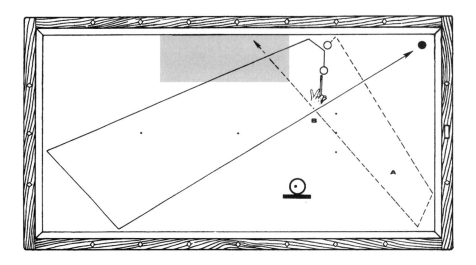

137 Three-rail position drive, short

The key in this pattern is to bank the white ball into the end rail. Position play like this always impresses people, but it isn't so tough when you consider the size of the acceptable target zone. There is a chance of a kiss at point B, but the chance is worth taking. If the cueball were at A to begin with, not enough speed could be given to the white to make it reach the shaded area. Best then would be to leave the white near the lower right corner and come up behind the red for the reason given in Diagram 139.

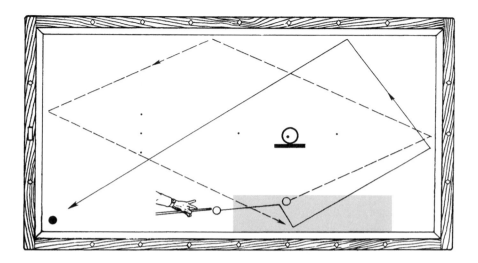

138 Three-rail position drive, long

The idea given in Diagram 136 won't quite work here, so hit the red full and use spin to establish the proper angle for the cueball off the first rail. The object ball banks three rails and enters the target zone as shown.

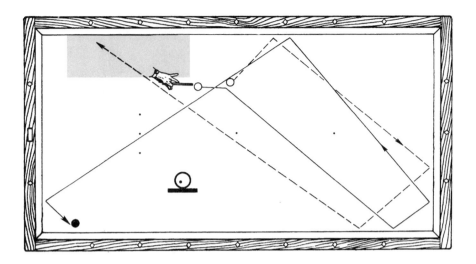

139 Another three-rail position drive

When the first ball can be brought to the same end as the second ball, there is almost bound to be another good shot if the cueball can be made to come up behind the second ball. In the diagrammed example, the next shot will either be a short angle off the left side of the white or a three- or five-railer off the left side of the red.

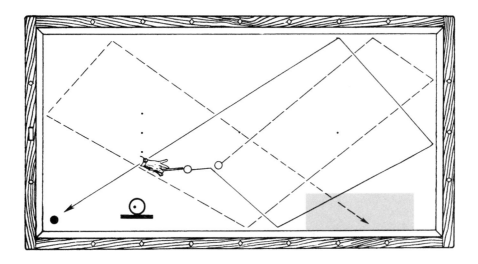

140 Five-rail position drive

When the patterns in Diagrams 136 and 138 don't look applicable, the one here can be tried. Even though the first ball is driven five rails, fabulous speed control isn't essential because of the generous size of the target zone.

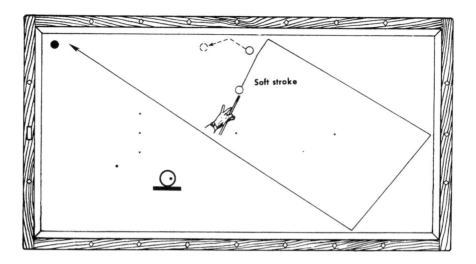

Soft stroke

141 One-rail position cut

Except for Diagram 139, the previous examples showed how to bring the first ball to a zone near the same long rail along which the point is scored. Here the first ball is already in a good place, so the idea is to keep it there. Cut the white very thin and use whatever English is needed to give the cueball the right angle off the first rail. Estimating the curve of the cueball as it rolls to the first ball is no problem when only a foot or two must be crossed. Position can also be played in shots of this general type by hitting the white full and banking it twice across.

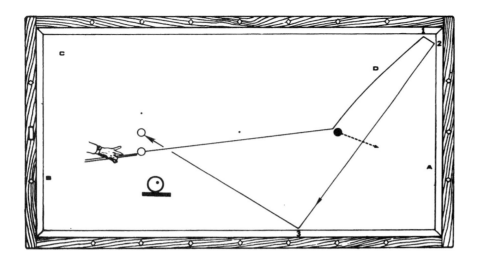

142 The opening break shot

Your objective on the opening break shot should be to bank the red to A, to the middle of the long rail, to B, and finally to the vicinity of D. If the cueball scores squarely on the white, the white will be knocked into the corner at C and there will be another natural shot. Raymond Ceulemans averages nearly three on the break.

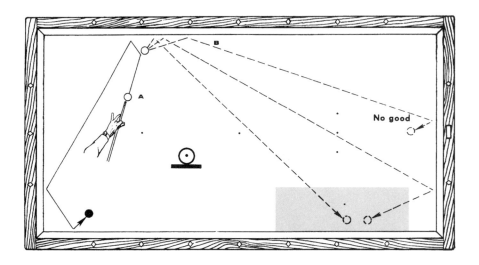

143 Full-hit short angle

A common error on short angles is to hit the first ball so thin that it comes to rest near the middle portion of the far short rail, a poor place for it as far as position play is concerned. Correct is to hit more ball and use less English so that the first ball enters the position zone along one of the two diagrammed paths. If the cue-ball is at A initially, shoot very softly with no English, driving the first ball no farther than B; you should be left a short angle off one ball or another. (This last idea is from the late Bud Harris of San Francisco, three-time United States champion.)

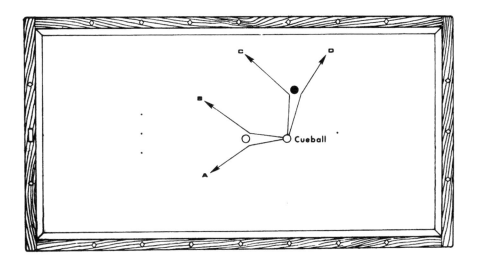

144 Center-of-the-table principle

There are at least six good shots that can be played in this position: three or five rails off the right side of the red, three or five rails off the right side of the white, or three rails off the left side of either ball. Which is best? Opinions differ, as you will discover if you seek any. Soft off the right side of the red, leaving the red ball near the letter C, is probably best for the purposes of position because all three balls will be left in the central area of the table. There is almost bound to be a decent option. (I was told this by Jay Bozeman, probably the best player never to be world champion, who played strong billiards well into his eighties. When he talks, both the author and the reader should listen.)

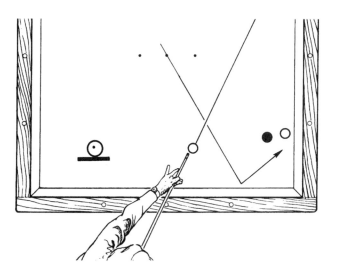

145 Extra-rail principle

When you plan to score on a ball or balls near a corner, it's best to play the shot four or five rails rather than three whenever possible. (See basic rule 6, page 346.)

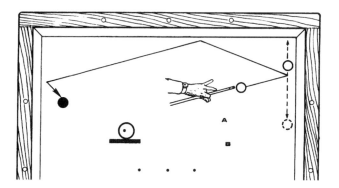

146 Thin-hit short angle

More from Bud Harris. If you hit the white ball softly and thin, you'll be left with another short angle. From point A, the first ball can still be held within three diamonds of the corner. From B it's best to use more speed and either try to leave the white at the lower right corner (out of the diagram) or to bank it all the way back to near its present location.

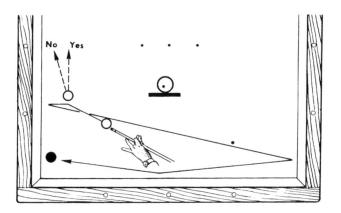

147 The parallel position principle

Why are the arrows labeled No and Yes? Because one leads to the unknown and the other to a good shot. If the white is sent along a course parallel to the side rail, it will be in a fine spot almost wherever it comes to rest. If the cueball lands gently on the red, in fact, the shooter will very likely have another position shot and a run of at least three. A dumb opponent will think it's luck.

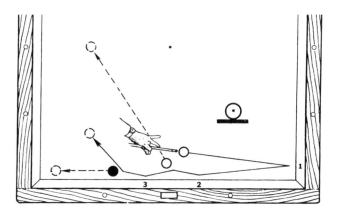

148 Back-up ticky position

Back-up tickys often turn out splendidly. Select a speed that is most likely to give the result shown.

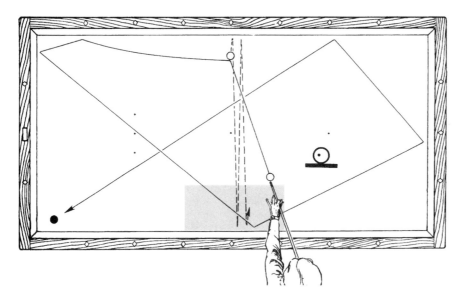

149 Cross-table position drive

If you can bank the white across the table three times, it will stop on the same side of the table as the other two balls and you'll have another good shot.

Still another new look at old shots

As St. Mark (patron saint of suckers) might have said, "What doth it profit a man to envision a long run and miss the first shot?" In other words, don't try to do too much too soon or you'll end up with a plethora of zeros on your scoresheet. As you become more confident and accurate you'll be able to attempt position on a wider range of shots. With that caveat, let's take a final look at a few earlier diagrams.

Diagram 10—Shooting softly will keep the first ball close to the side rail. If the position is such that the first ball must be hit fuller, it can sometimes be banked twice across for position.

Diagram 16, right—In shots a little easier than this one, it is sometimes worth it to hit a little more red ball in an attempt to angle it closer to the upper long rail.

Diagram 34—With a thin hit, adjust the speed to leave the white ball near the upper long rail. If the angle is such that a fuller hit is required, it is sometimes possible to bank the white three times across.

Diagram 135—Aside from the chance of a kiss, this is an excellent position shot. Practice it until you can leave the white ball near the upper long rail.

8

fifty selected shots
from master play

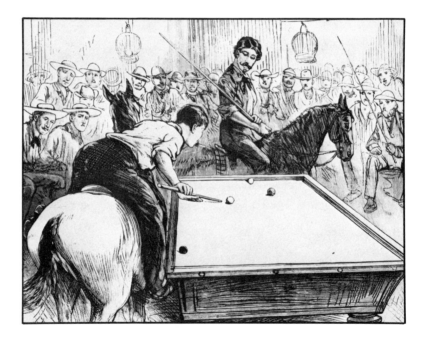

More horsing around, in California.
(*Illustrated Police News*, 1887)

What do the world's billiard grand masters do when confronted with a tough shot? They use their imaginations, their remarkable accuracy and control of speed, their deep understanding of cueball behavior, their uncanny banking judgment, and their knowledge of certain shots and stratagems. I can help you with the last part. In this section are fifty ways of getting out of tight spots taken from a notebook kept during thirty-five years of tournament competition.

Another thing the grand masters often do on tough shots is miss. During the course of a game they will usually miss a shot for every one they make. That's a pleasant feature of three-cushion: It's no disgrace to miss. In pool, if you don't make everything you go for, you're a bum.

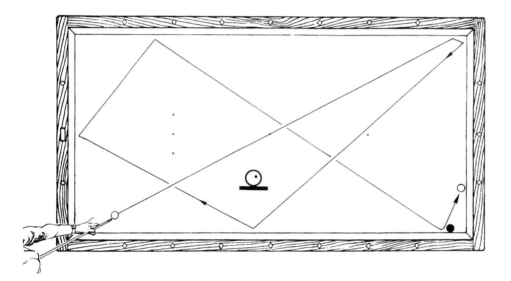

150 Six rails first

Watch for this avenue of approach to two balls in the corner.

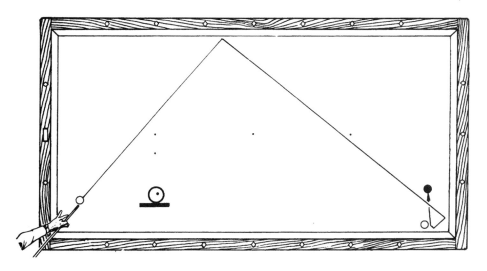

151 Into-the-corner natural bank

Often overlooked in favor of the five-rail bank. This is better because most players have fairly good accuracy at banking a ball into a corner.

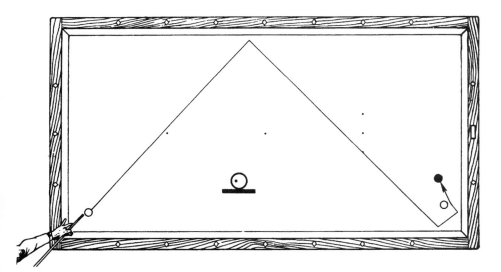

152 Reverse bank

Shooting from the corner into the middle of the opposite long rail with maximum reverse English puts the cueball on the path shown here . . . on my table. Find out what happens on yours and experiment with how much the path shifts when the aiming point is moved an inch or two to the left.

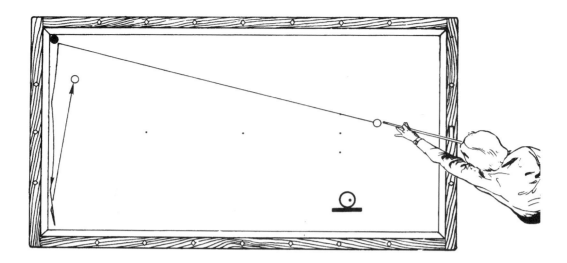

153 Kiss-across double-the-rail

What else is there? Might as well try this and get a standing ovation if it goes. If you can just get the cueball to kiss away to the left there are several scoring paths.

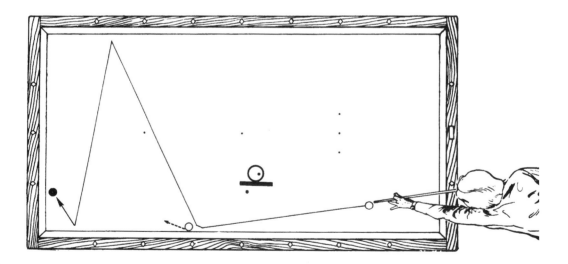

154 Rail-first running reverse

Tyros seldom think of using running English on this rail-first shot. The English on the second rail is "wrong-way" or hold-up. If the ball is still spinning when it reaches the third rail there will be a satisfying spurt into the point.

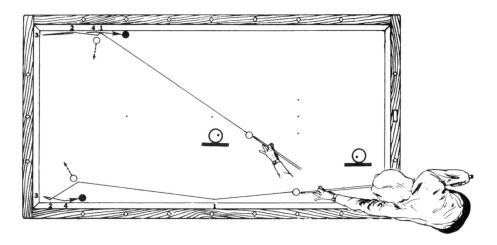

155 Two severe hold-up tickys

Both of these shots follow the same pattern—rail-first to one ball, then double-the-rail to the other, though the fourth rail isn't needed. The upper shot is often easier than a back-up ticky (Diagram 40) when the angle of approach is more than, say, 30 degrees. In the lower shot it is almost always better to go back to the side rail off the ball instead of straight into the end rail.

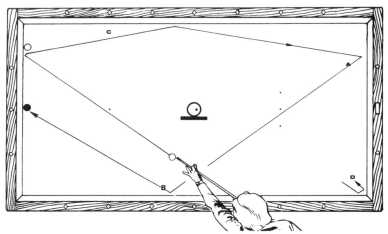

156 End rail first

This can be the best pattern to adopt when the second ball is in its diagrammed position or at A, B, C, or even D. Backing out of the corner to hit a ball at D is an eight-rail shot and on a slow table takes a King Kong stroke. In aiming the eight-railer, squirt has to be taken into account (Diagram 108).

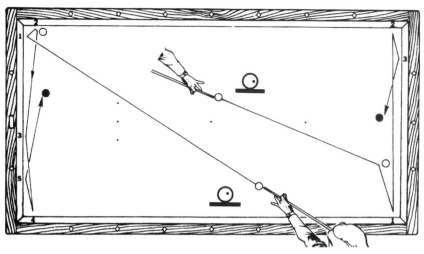

157 Snap-back double-the-rail

Once you get the hang of shots like these you may never go back to pool. Both, sometimes, make off four rails instead of five and three as drawn. I call the one at the right a reverse cross-table spin-out.

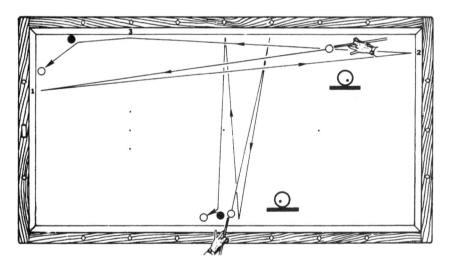

158 Up-and-down draw bank

Nabih Yousri, the former Egyptian champion from Cairo, who now lives in exotic Vallejo, California, is a devotee of the up-and-down draw bank. A cross-table version is also shown. Use enough speed to make sure the draw English works off the first rail.

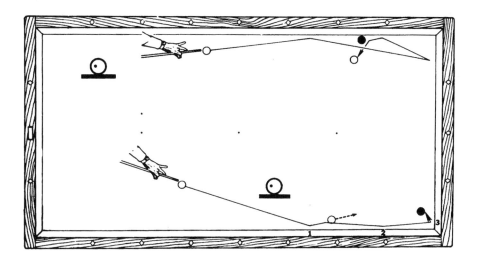

159 Above-the-ball double-the-rail

The shot at the top is a lovely thing. I made it once in winning a match against Miss Noriko Katsura of Tokyo during one of her visits to California. She won the next game, but for a minute there I was Ladies' Champion of Japan.

(Noriko was also *Men's* Champion of Japan in a four-ball version of straight billiards that is popular there. She and her older sister Masako have proven that women can play world-class billiards if they choose to fling themselves into it the way men do.)

The little-known follow ticky

At the bottom, there seems to be no way to keep the cueball close enough to the rail on a ticky pattern with such a little hole to go through. The secret lies in hitting the rail farther from the ball than on a standard ticky and following through the white ball. I learned this shot from San Francisco's Jimmie Lee, now long gone, who at age eighty still played a hell of a game.

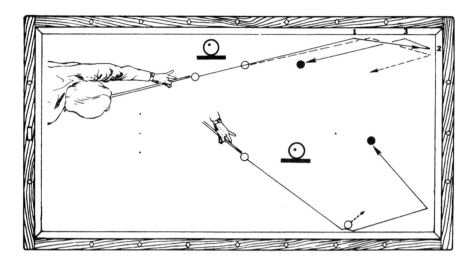

160 Force-follow double-the-rail

If you've got a good follow stroke and the cueball is not far from the first ball, the shot at the top is quite practical.

Force-through ticky

At the bottom, a ticky doesn't seem possible because the hole is too small to pass the cueball. The trick is to shoot firmly so that the cueball sinks into the rubber enough to squeeze through. The action sometimes occurs by accident on rail-first shots that are stroked with speed.

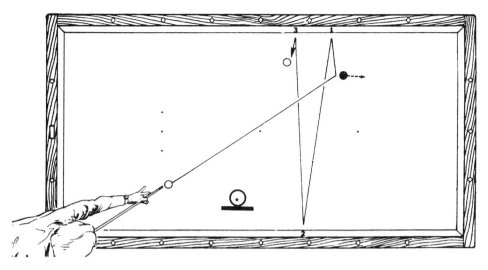

161 The world champion's uphill cross-table

When Raymond Ceulemans made this unorthodox shot in the 1966 world tournament, I saw an old-timer frown and mutter, "That shot ain't in the book."

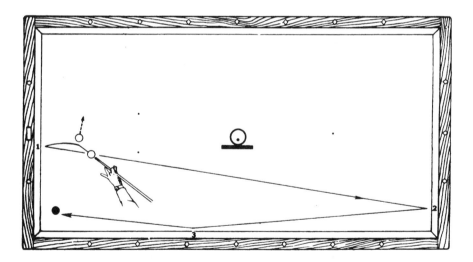

162 Up-and-down draw shot

The white must be cut thinner than is comfortable to keep it from banking into the red. Draw pulls it back into a scoring path.

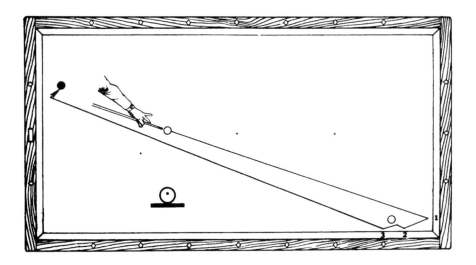

163 Back-up ticky extended

Not a bad choice when the red is big. It sometimes requires the subtleties explained in Diagrams 89 and 90.

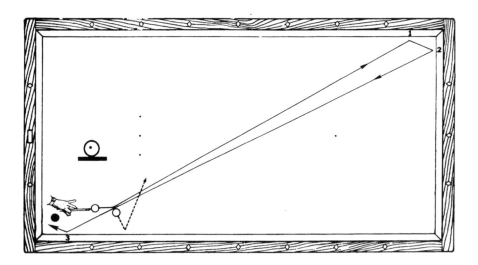

164 Long-angle hold-up

Use a little hold-up English. A tough shot to judge accurately.

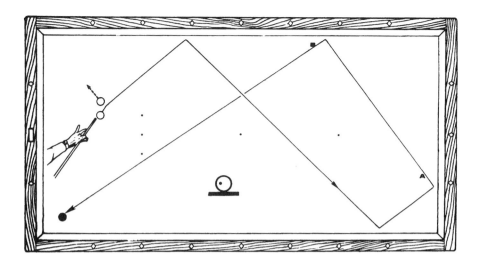

165 Reverse around the table

Because reverse English tends to kill cueball speed, plenty of power is needed on this shot to get all the way around the table. It's not so bad, though, when the first ball can be hit thin, as here. The pattern also comes into consideration when the second ball is at A or B or points between.

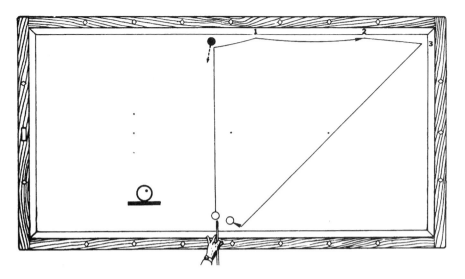

166 Kobayashi's back-to-the-rail shot

In the 1974 world tournament in Belgium, this position came up for Nobuaki Kobayashi, many times champion of Japan. Twice he bent over and aimed with high English off the left side of the red, and twice he straightened up, fearful of banking the red across the table into the white. He finally played it as diagrammed. It missed by a hair, but it was a great idea. He won the tournament by a single point, running six and out in the final game against Ceulemans in one of the most dramatic games ever played.

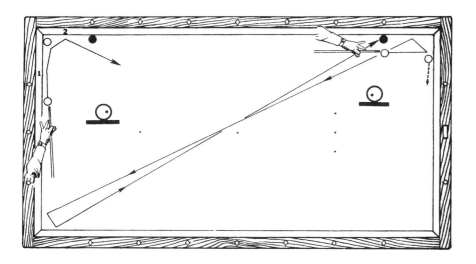

167 The short four-railer

Consider these patterns when the hit on the red seems too tough. The cueball can be made to return to the long rail even farther from the corner than the first diamond. The rail-first version at the upper left requires a thin hit on the white to avoid a kiss.

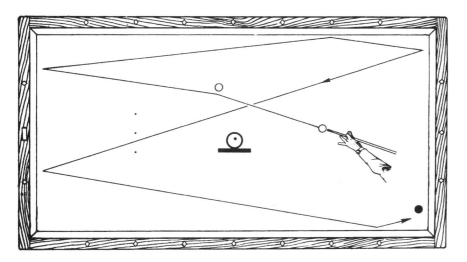

168 Adolfo Suarez and his flying W

Adolfo Suarez, the colorful 1961 world champion from Peru, had an aggressive style of play and a powerful stroke. One of his trademarks was the so-called flying W. It may not look like much on paper, but in fact it is extremely difficult.

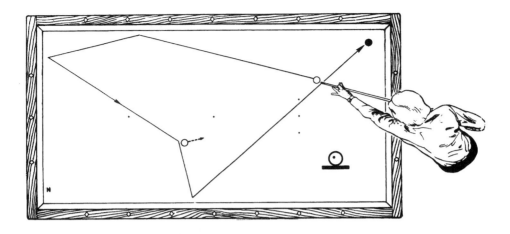

169 Around-the-table umbrella

Related to the standard umbrella (Diagram 54), but tougher. The system can help.
Estimate the point the cueball will hit on the second rail, then draw a line from there
to the side of the white ball, extending it to learn the required third-rail number.
Some players in the diagrammed predicament would try to follow straight through
the white ball with high left, hoping for a first-rail contact at N and a third-rail contact near the red, a shot that is good when the cueball is closer to the white.

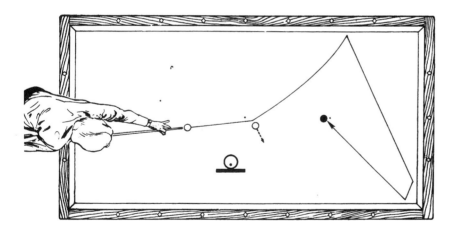

170 Hook draw

There are several nasty banks you can try in this terrible position, but they are no
easier than the hook draw diagrammed. Use plenty of draw and no English. If not
too much speed is used, the white can be cut thinner than you might expect.

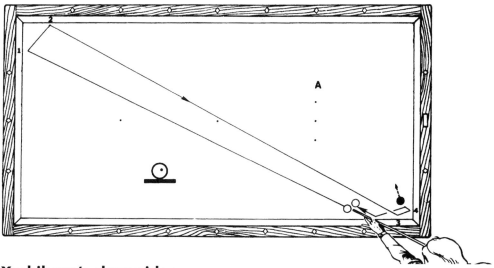

171 Yoshihara's clever idea

Another shot from the 1974 world tournament, this time with Japan's brilliant young Yoshio Yoshihara at the table. He scored the point as shown, coming into the corner short to back off the red into the white. Remember this method of approaching two balls in the corner on standard banks from cueball positions like A. The corner is easy to find—just come in a little short.

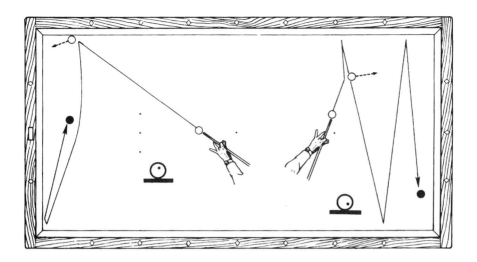

172 Cross-table swing

At the left, a high ball and a little right English will make the cueball "swing" around the red and back out to score.

Three-times-across walk-down

At the right, the cueball, because of reverse English on the second rail, tends to straighten out and go back and forth at right angles to the long rails. A slightly elevated cue encourages the cueball to keep working its way toward the red. Use enough speed to count off the fourth rail if it misses off the third. A rule to remember: On any two-way shot, always shoot hard enough to score the second way.

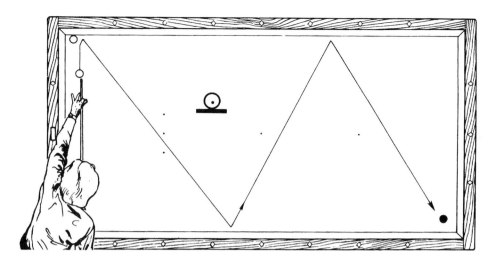

173 Double zigzag

You've got to try this a few times to get a feeling for the angle.

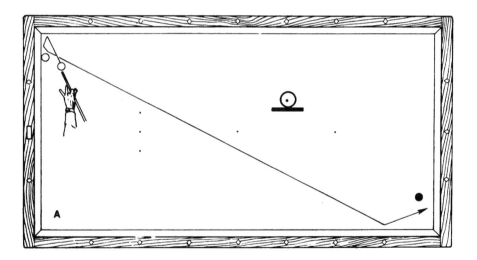

174 Two rails first out of the corner

A soft stroke is all that's needed. With a thinner hit on the white, the cueball can be sent all around the table to score on a red ball at A. Not very often, though.

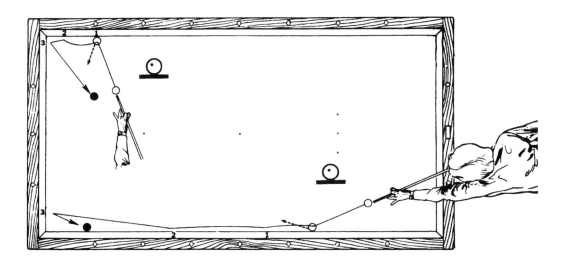

175 Smash-through spin-out

At the upper left is a variation of Diagram 94. From a steep angle of approach like this a surprisingly sharp spin-out is possible off the third rail.

Force-follow spin-back

The shot along the lower rail, which occasionally comes up in practical play, is pretty enough to use in an exhibition of trick shots.

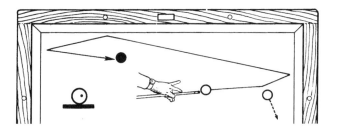

176 Hold-up flat short angle

There is no way to make this short angle with no English or running English. You must use hold-up and shoot firmly enough so that it still has "bite" on the third rail.

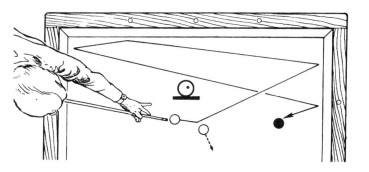

177 Hold-up flat short angle extended

A longer version of the previous shot. The red is actually a big ball in this pattern because if you miss it on the approach, you'll make it on the rebound. Johann Scherz of Austria, several times champion of Europe, takes hardly more than one second to aim this shot.

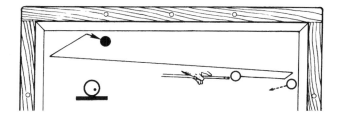

178 Inside cross-table reverse

Don't baby this. Some speed is needed to give the cueball the proper draw action off the first rail and spin off the second.

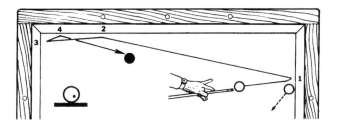

179 Cross-table through-the-hole reverse

If the second ball isn't in the right position for the previous pattern, you can sometimes send the cueball through the hole to back out and score. The fourth rail isn't needed.

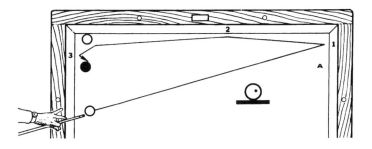

180 Hold-up cross-table bank

Hitting point A with no English is possible (Diagram 51), but it would take a delicate hit on the white to permit the cueball to touch the third rail before the red. Hitting the first rail closer to the corner as shown and using a little hold-up English provides a better angle of approach to the white.

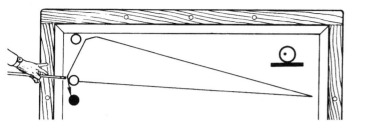

181 Angled cross-table bank

Here the object balls are too far apart for the normal Diagram 51 treatment. In order to come in on the white at an angle that provides some chance of scoring, hit the first rail farther from the corner, compensating with English.

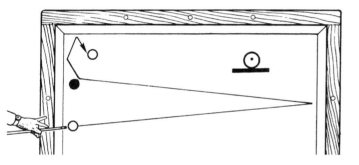

182 Cross-table corner back-out

I would hate to have to shoot this for the rent. Use no English and try to hit half the red ball. Soft stroke.

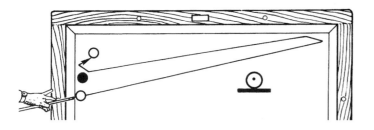

183 A Gus Copulos specialty

Gus Copulos was one of the great players of the 1920s and one of the developers of the diamond system. Only a player of his gifts would think of a shot like this. It's not difficult once you get the idea. From the second diamond it's very nearly impossible.

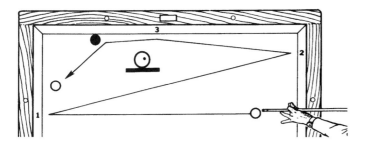

184 Twice-across end-rail bank

A good player might make this two out of three times.

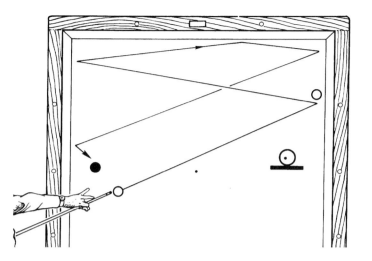

185 Back-around short angle

Not enough left English can be put on the cueball to make this shot as a standard short angle, so this unusual pattern can be tried. Bill Hynes, 1969 United States champion, had very good judgment on this shot and could convince you that it's practical.

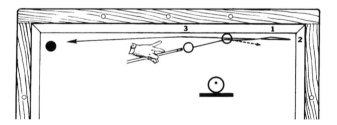

186 Stay-on-the-rail smash-through

Keeping the cueball close to the end rail on a force follow like this is not easy. Use only the slightest hint of left English, just enough to give the cueball the proper flat angle off the second rail. The cueball should be rolling without English when it hits the red.

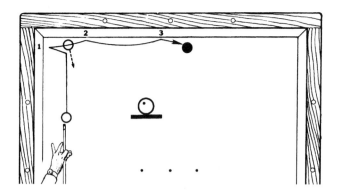

187 Reverse follow back-to-the-rail

This fancy shot is almost a cinch in the given position. Use left English as well as high follow and shoot fairly hard. If you've never seen this one, ask a good player to demonstrate it.

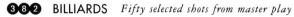

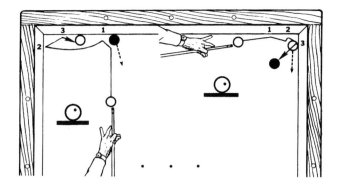

188 Snake around a ball

The snake shot at the left is not for beginners. A lot of high right English is needed along with as full a hit on red as possible, but not much speed. At the Cushion and Cue in Oak Park, Michigan, I saw Larry "Boston Shorty" Johnson make it against Chicago's Luis Campos.

Kiss ticky

At the right, a standard ticky won't work because the white will kiss the red away. There's a subtlety that solves the problem. Hit the rail first and land full enough on the white to get a double-kiss. The kiss forces the white through the hole while the cueball gets two more rails in the corner before hitting the red. I wish I could give credit to the inventor of this ingenious play, but his name is lost in the swirling mists of yesteryear.

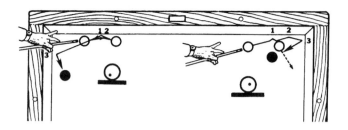

189 Ball-first ticky

This is the kind of thing I learned by hanging around with Jimmie Lee and Bud Harris at the long-gone Palace Billiards in San Francisco. At the right, the hole is so small that the cueball in a normal ticky pattern will tend to spin too much off the third rail unless hard-to-judge hold-up is used. But by first hitting the white thin on the left, the hole is enlarged before the ticky pattern begins! The cueball goes off the white to the rail and gets back to the white before the white is completely out of the way. *Then* the cueball gets two more rails in the corner. Can sometimes be used to miss a kiss when the kiss ticky in the previous diagram is too hard to judge.

Rail-first corner draw

The shot at the left is not only difficult, but—like the kiss ticky and the ball-first ticky—when you make it everybody is liable to say you didn't. The cueball hits the rail first, then the white, then draws back to the end rail before going to the side rail. The action is sometimes too fast for the eye to follow.

what's the best shot?

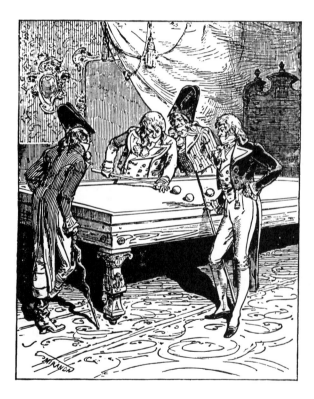

In revolutionary France.
(*Modern Billiards*, 1881)

Here are two dozen test positions to exercise your brain. Answers and brief discussion are given following Diagram 209. You might disagree with my conclusions, which is perfectly all right with me. Maybe the *Reader's Digest* will someday run diagrams like these with trips to Belgium offered to those who reply correctly.

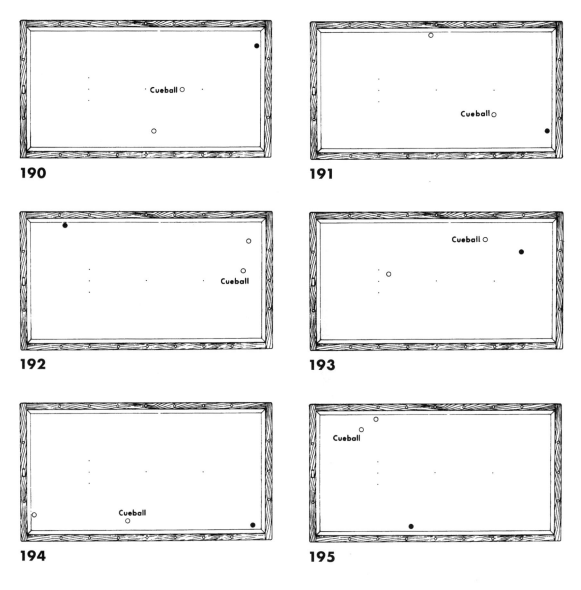

190

191

192

193

194

195

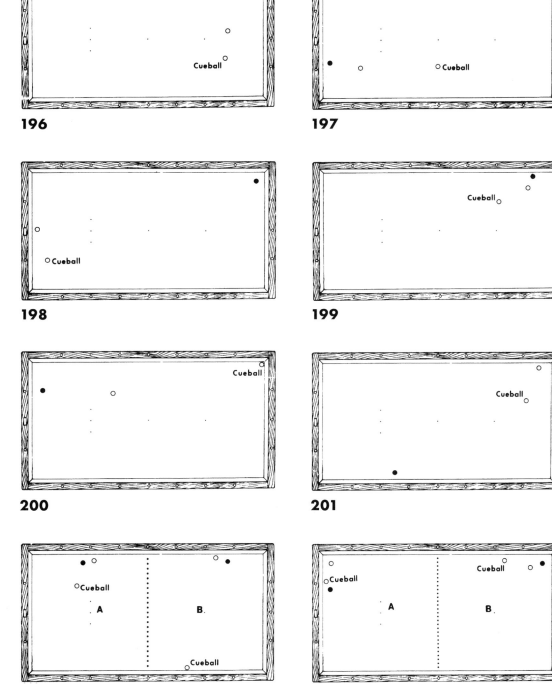

196

197

198

199

200

201

202

203

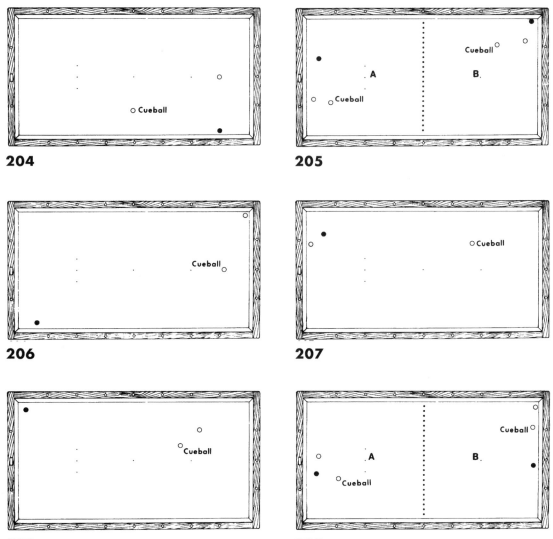

204

205

206

207

208

209

Answers to "What's the best shot?"

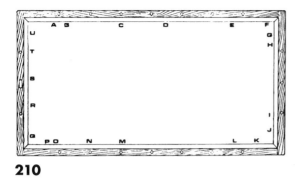

210

190—Left-hand English a hair below center off the right side of the white ball. Strike rails at Q, P, and E. (The letters in all of the answers refer to Diagram 210.) Like Diagram 30, but without the curved path to the first rail.

191—Go off the left side of the white with no English and slight follow. Hit rails at C, U, and L.

192—Three possibilities. Safest is an outside zigzag, hitting rails at E, M, and T (Diagram 9). Other good shots are the inside zigzag (G, F, M, T), rather like Diagram 10. Then there is the side rail first off the red with no English (compare Diagrams 53 and 93).

193—If safety doesn't concern you, shoot a plus system shot off the right side of the red (Diagram 76). Safer and only slightly more difficult is the long-angle drop-in off the right side of the white (T, E, G).

194—You can go off the right side of the white to C and J or K, or you can try the pattern in Diagram 53. Best is off the left side of the white with high left English, hitting rails at Q, P, and D, which makes use of the red as a big ball.

195—The Diagram 29 pattern can be used off either ball.

196—Variations of 9, 10, 24, and 85 can be weighed in positions like this. A beautiful possibility is the reverse shot off the left side of the white. Use heavy right English, make roughly a half-ball hit on the white, and try for the rails at D, O, and Q.

197—The balls are in an unfriendly attitude for banks, so you might as well try a reverse cross-table off the left side of the white with low left, trying for rails at O, A, and S. Check Diagrams 31 and 32.

198—The diagonal draw (Diagram 7) is better here than the outside zigzag (Diagram 9) for reasons of safety.

199—Best is the bank—D, T, M, H, red ball, side rail, white ball.

200—The only chance is a five-rail bank—N, R, C, I, L, white, red. An unusual feature is that the cueball passes between the balls on the way to the third rail.

201—A ticky behind the red is possible, and so is a corner plunge (Diagram 30). A good shot is softly off the right side of the white, banking it out of the way of a kiss, trying for rails at G, F, and M. If the white ends up near L, you are set for another good shot and are safe if you miss. There is more in this position. With the same hit on the white but with follow instead of left, the cueball can be made to hit the second rail at E and the third at S, coming in on the red from behind.

202—Shot A: The white is big, so play a five-rail shot off the right side of the red. Shoot hard, use right English and enough follow to make the cueball bend into the long rail at about D.
   Shot B: Five rails first—A, U, M, H, E, red, white.

203—Shot A: If doubling-the-rail off white looks tough there is sometimes the easy option of shooting straight into the long rail with left English, getting two rails in the corner, hitting the white, then back to the short rail before the red.
   Shot B: You can double the long rail, contacting it first at B, you can play a plus system shot by shooting into Q, or you can try a hold-up ticky off the red. There is also a good two-rails-first snap-back shot. Shoot crisply into the corner with no English, hitting the long rail first at F. The cueball comes almost straight off the end rail into the side of the red, then goes back to the long rail near F and rebounds off at a steep angle into the white. If you ever see me hanging around, I'll demonstrate it.

204—Five rails off the left side of the white. The first part of the pattern is given in Diagram 105.

205—Shot A: A high-percentage shot is the double-the-rail draw off the right side of the white with maximum left English (Diagram 18).

Shot B: Several kinds of banks can be tried here, but I currently believe that the least difficult one is a long version of the two-rail-first pattern given in Diagram 51. No English.

206—You could play a rail-first (off the red) short angle extended à la Diagram 93, but a safer shot is rail-first to the right side of the white, getting a second rail at F, then proceeding down the table diagonally toward the red in search of a third rail. To go short like this, use no English, contrary to what I said about Diagram 201, in which the ball is hit first. Here, English makes the cueball go long because it spins off the second rail. If the red ball is near the end rail at S, for example, English is needed. Shoot softly for safety.

207—Give your opponent credit for having left you safe. Return the favor by going off the right side of the white with draw and no English. The cueball may go four rails to score or it may go in short and back up off the sixth rail at U to score. If it does neither, which is likely, the other cueball is far down the table and your opponent is in the same pickle you were.

208—Feather the left side of the white with extreme right English and a soft stroke. The spin will add speed to the cueball off the first rail to carry it around the table. There is no kiss if the white is hit extremely thin so that it doesn't go anyplace.

With the cueball an inch or two to the right, a force follow through the white with high right, hitting the first rail near E, is a possibility.

209—Shot A: Twice across off the white, hitting the first rail near A. *Use follow only* to make the cueball bend slightly toward the red as it crosses the table toward the second rail at P. The cueball is supposed to score after it hits one or two more side rails.

Shot B: A tough one in conclusion. On fast equipment I might try the reverse around-the-table shot off the red, as in Diagram 165, especially if the white is big in the corner. Otherwise there is a cross-table shot off the left side of the white with low right English in the manner of Diagram 17.

glossary

Balkline—A version of straight billiards made more difficult by drawing lines on the cloth across which balls must be driven. Once very popular in the United States, still played in Europe and Japan.

Diamonds—Small spots or discs set into the wooden part of the rails that can be used as aids in calculating certain shots. They haven't been shaped like diamonds since about 1910, but the name has persisted. The word is also used as a measure of distance, one diamond equaling fourteen inches on a standard five-foot-wide table.

Elevation—Raising the butt of the cue in order to hit the cueball at a downward angle.

First object ball—The ball the cueball hits first. Can be either the red or the white.

Second object ball—The ball the cueball hits second.

Head of table—The end of the table where the cueball is placed at the start of the game. The end of the table where the nameplate is, if there is one.

Hold-up—English that tends to make the ball slow down when it hits a rail.

Hold-up makes the angle of rebound greater than the angle of approach.

Kissed in—A shot is said to be kissed in when a point is made because of an accidental collision or collisions.

Kissed out—A shot is said to be kissed out when it fails to score because of an accidental collision or collisions.

Long roll, short roll—A ball rolling diagonally across the table from corner to corner is said to be rolling long if it curves toward the end rail and away from the side rail. When rolling short it bends toward the side rail. If the table is level, if the balls are round, if the cloth has nap and is oriented properly, balls will roll long at the head of the table, short at the foot. The best billiard cloths today, such as the top grades made by Simonis of Belgium and Gorina of Spain, have no significant nap. Fine, fast cloth is a must.

Nameplate—A metal plate carrying the manufacturer's name set into the center of one end rail on many billiard tables. Used for short instead of the phrase "the center of the head rail."

Natural—A natural shot is one that can be made with natural (running) English, without forcing the cueball to curve, and in which each rail contacted is adjacent to the previous one. Loosely, any easy, obvious, or straightforward shot.

Natural English—See Running English. The spin a ball naturally picks up when it rolls into a rail at an angle is natural English.

Rail—The cushion or rubber that lines the field of play. "Stuck on the gum" means frozen to a cushion.

Reverse—Extreme hold-up. Sometimes taken to mean draw, but not in this book.

Running English—Spin that makes the cueball speed up when it hits a rail.

Running English makes the angle of rebound smaller than the angle of approach. Also called natural English (see above). Usually applied with the tip above center.

Scratch—A point scored in a manner other than the one intended.

Straight billiards—A form of the game suitable for beginners and experts alike in which a point is scored merely by hitting the two object balls with the cueball. Also called straight rail.

Time shot—An intentional kiss-in, a shot in which the player deliberately sets all three balls in motion.

appendixes

book one—POOL

Where to go for more information

After decades of relative inactivity, authors and publishers awoke in the 1990s and began turning out books about the game at a record pace. Reviews of sixteen of them can be found in *Byrne's Wonderful World of Pool and Billiards* (1996).

Players interested in trick shots should check the last pages of *Byrne's Treasury of Trick Shots in Pool and Billiards* (1982), where capsule reviews can be found of thirteen books, including those by Mingaud (1830), Phelan (1858), McCleery (1890), Thatcher (1898), Herrmann (1902), and Hood (1918), as well as more recent titles.

Everybody should own a copy of the most recent *Official Rules & Records Book* published by the Billiard Congress of America, 910 23rd Avenue, Coralville, IA.

To see what's available, check new and used bookstores, billiard supply stores, libraries, the billiard trade magazines, and the catalogs published by such mail-order companies as Billiard Library (800-245-5542) and Mueller Sporting Goods (800-925-7665).

Three national periodicals are devoted to the game of pool. Sample copies are yours if you send five dollars for postage and handling to:

Billiards Digest, 122 South Michigan Avenue, Suite 1506, Chicago, IL 60603
Pool and Billiard Magazine, P.O. Box 1515, Summerville, SC 29484
The National Billiard News, Box 807, Northville, MI 48167

There are a fluctuating number of local and regional pool magazines and newsletters. Ask your billiard retailer or local tavern league secretary if there are any in your area.

For information on amateur and professional tournaments, phone:

Billiard Congress of America—319-351-2112
National 9-ball Tour—972-712-TOUR
Mali Florida Tour—561-743-9501
Steve Mizerak Senior Tour—407-840-0048
Professional Cuesports Association—214-553-8082
Pro Billiard Tour—352-596-7808
Women's Professional Billiard Association—714-252-4789
American Poolplayers Association—3-RACK-EM
Valley National Eight-ball Association—517-892-4536
National Wheelchair Billiards Association—216-281-8536

A huge change since this book's debut in 1978 is the plethora of videotapes available now in billiard stores or by mail. There are dozens of how-to-play tapes featuring various champions and teachers, some of them only slightly better than home-movie quality, others quite nicely produced. Professionally produced with two cameras and two commentators are the tapes of pool tournament matches available from Accu-Stats Video Productions, Box 299, Bloomingdale, NJ 07403. Call 800-828-0397 for a free thirty-two-page catalog.

My own series of six videotapes was produced on Hollywood sound stages by Premiere Home Video, 755 North Highland, Hollywood, CA 90038 (800-525-4998). A brief look at the contents:

Rack 'em Up! The world of pool—cue making, slate mining, cloth weaving, tournaments, rules of games, tips on how to handle a cue and how to aim, a tour of a well-stocked billiard supply store, and a look at how a pro player breaks the balls and runs the table.

Byrne's Standard Video of Pool, Vol. I and Vol. II—A comprehensive course on playing pool from the fundamentals to advanced spin, swerve, jump, and massé shots, taped with the aid of three cameras, close-ups, slow motion, and computer graphics.

Byrne's Standard Video of Trick Shots, Vol. III and Vol. IV—Eighty trick shots within the reach of intermediate players, plus a few eye-popping showstoppers. Most of the shots depend more on secret information than fabulous skill.

Byrne's Power Pool Workout, Vol. V. Practice methods and drills designed to shorten learning time for students willing to work.

See also the Internet references at the end of the next appendix.

book two—BILLIARDS

Where to go for more information

Readers interested in watching or playing in a three-cushion tournament, or who simply want to support the grand old game and keep in touch with what's going on, should join the United States Billiard Association. The USBA sends out a monthly newsletter that lists forthcoming tournaments—there are fifteen or twenty a year—and gives the results of recent events. For a sample copy and information, write to:

Bob Jewett, Secretary
U.S. Billiard Association
962 Stony Hill Road
Redwood City, CA 94061

Of the three national magazines listed in the appendix to Book One, only *Billiards Digest* covers three-cushion, reporting on major tournaments, and occasionally running an instructional article. For international coverage of the game, which is very popular in Europe, there is *World Report 3-Cushion,* which is published in English eleven times a year. For subscription information, write to the magazine at P.O. Box 30166, 3001 DD Rotterdam, The Netherlands.

For videotapes of matches between the world's greatest players, see the catalog available from Accu-Stats Video Productions (800-828-0397). Watch the trick-shot show by Turkey's sensational Semih Sayginer and you'll be hooked. Also delicious are any of the low-inning games by Blomdahl.

English-speaking students looking for printed three-cushion instruction have a limited choice once they've devoured the billiard sections of my own books. Copies of Willie Hoppe's hoary classic *Billiards As It Should Be Played* (1941, with several later reprints) can sometimes be found on the secondhand market, and there are the technical works on diamond systems described at the end of *Byrne's Wonderful World of Pool and Billiards*. Eddie Robin's exhaustive (and exhausting!) *Position Play in Three-Cushion Billiards* (1979) is available by writing Billiard World Publishing, Box 12417, Las Vegas, NV 89112-0417. Two 1998 titles from the same publisher are *500 Essential Shots of 3-Cushion Billiards* and *500 Advanced Shots of 3-Cushion Billiards*.

And leave us not forget the fast-growing and fast-changing Internet. For those of you who are logged on, use your search engine to find references to "billiards." ("Pool" might get you more than you wanted to know about swimming.) If you know how to access news groups, an interesting one is rec.sport.billiard

Want to play Equal Offense (see Rules of Major Pool Games) in real time against players all over the world? You'll need a pool table, a few teammates, and a computer. Log on to the International Equal Offense home page at http://www.bca-pool.com/ieo/

Other billiard links can be found on the home page of the Billiard Congress of America at http://www.bca-pool.com

Here are some others worth checking out:

http://www.billiardsdigest.com
www.poolmag.com
www.carom.com
www.billiardworld.com
www.accessone.com/~mavlon
www.interactive.line.com/~ira/billiard.html
www.tourboard.com
www.fhi-berlin.mpg.de/~unger/glossary.html
www.mueller-sporting-goods.com/
www.accu-stats.com
www.ifi.uio.no/~hermunda/snooker
www.poolplayers.com/
www.billiards.cso.uiuc.edu/billiards/tv/espn
www.csj.net/~deilerin/vpool/index.htm

indexes

book one—POOL

See also the table of contents

book two—BILLIARDS

See also the table of contents